The Winning Factor

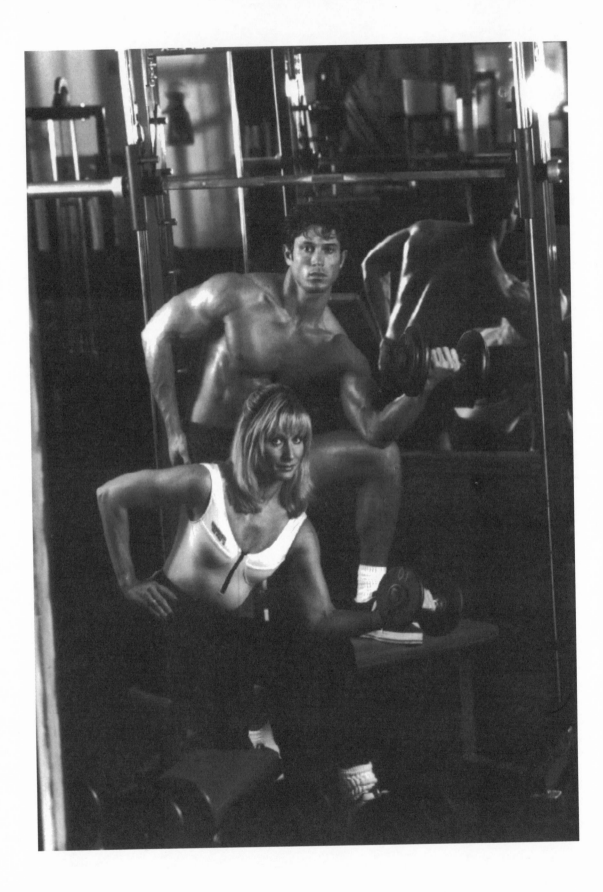

The Winning Factor

Ultimate Fitness Experience for Everyone

John Schaeffer, M.F.S., S.S.C., S.P.N.

with **Anthony Clark**

M. Evans and Company, Inc. • *New York*

M. Evans and Company, Inc.
216 East 49th Street
New York, New York 10017

Library of Congress Cataloging-in-Publication Data

Schaeffer, John.
    The winning factor : ultimate fitness experience for everyone /
John Schaeffer with Anthony Clark.
        p.   cm.
    ISBN 0-87131-845-8 (pbk.)
    1. Bodybuilding.   2. Weight training   3. Physical fitness.
I. Clark, Anthony.   II. Title.
GV546.S33   1998
613.7'1—dc21   97-44970

Design and composition by John Reinhardt Book Design

Manufactured in the United States of America

9 8 7 6 5 4 3 2 1

As we travel through life, we experience the good and the bad that the world has to offer, and we can only hope our lives have molded to become the type of person who will influence the people we come in touch with positively.

Through my life; those family, friends, and one-time acquaintances who left a lasting impact on the development of my character must all have a share in the dedication of this book.

It has been through experiences in life that I have become the person I am. I can only hope to be an asset to the small space I occupy in this world, and in some way give something to you from my experiences that may positively influence your life. No matter what your life's experience is, it is your choice to become the type of person you choose to be.

No one can ever change that but you!

John Schaeffer

Acknowledgments

A special thanks to Frederick Carl Hatfield, Ph.D., and I.S.S.A. (the International Sports Sciences Association). I.S.S.A., in my opinion, is head and shoulders above the field of fitness certification. I am honored to be affiliated with Dr. Hatfield and I.S.S.A. Anyone interested in I.S.S.A. certifications can contact them at 1-800-892-4772.

Also, a special thanks to D. J. Reeves and Dr. Fred Bell for all their assistance. And last, but not least, to (the Big Man) Anthony Clark, who helped make this book possible.

Images by

Studio 518 Photography
Allan Schaeffer, Photographer
48 East Mountain Avenue
Robesonia, PA 19551
(610) 693-5181
STUDIO_518@prodigy.net

Weight Training

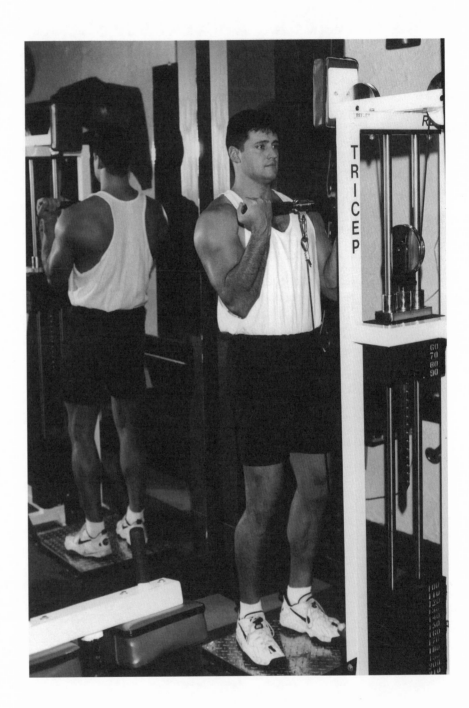

Chapter One

Weight Training

We've often read about major-league baseball players or professional football players who make weight training an important part of their fitness routine. More recently, though, there has been a definite increase of people in general who go regularly to a gym to lift weights. In 1998, the Associated Press alerted its readers that weight training is "emerging as a prescription for twenty-first century living."

However, as the owner-operator of a gym in eastern Pennsylvania, I get people from all walks of life. Many of them still come in with an inaccurate picture of what exactly weight training is, or how it can help them in their own fitness program. The truth is, despite its growing popularity, lifting weights is still often looked on as something extreme, almost dangerous. I can only compare this idea to a similar notion that once existed about people who put on rubber-soled shoes and funny-looking shorts to go out running in the streets, where they were even pelted with abuse occasionally. The notion that weight lifting is something radical, or only for athletes, will, believe me, one day seem as quaint as the old ideas about running do now. If anything, going by what I've seen, the chances of dramatic changes for the better are higher, and the risks of injury lower, for most people who only weight-train than for those who only run. One of the things this book will do for you is show you the best way to set up an exercise program so you get the benefits of an aerobic exercise like running along with the anaerobic benefits of weight training.

Almost all of the concerns people express about getting involved in weight training seem to be summed up under the word "muscle-bound." If you are worried about this, let me reassure you in the strongest terms possible that weight training will not make you a victim of muscles that swell up out of control. Equally, weight training will not make you stiff or slow. It will not slow down your reflexes. Many research studies have proven that the opposite of these worries is what actually happens. Weight training increases your speed and enhances your coordination at the same time it makes you stronger. This is the reason so many athletes lift weights regularly.

It is also important to know that as an essential, completely natural part of the training process itself, you are in control. You set the goals on how you want to look when you start a weight training program. Let's try to understand a little about how all this happens by looking at just what weight training is.

When you take a dumbbell in your hand and pull it toward your shoulder, you contract the bundles of muscle fibers that form the biceps at the front of your upper arm. As you straighten the arm out while holding the dumbbell, it is the triceps at the back of your upper arm that contract. This apparently simple movement by your arm actually requires a complex series of inner movements and adjustments by tendons, muscles, bones, and bursae. However, the muscle fibers inside the bundles making up biceps and triceps can only contract, and they do this by contracting in ordered unison as they work against the weight and resistance of the dumbbell to raise and lower it.

If the dumbbell is heavy enough and you ask your arm to raise and lower it enough times, a very interesting thing happens. The small muscle fibers that have been contracting in concert begin to develop tiny tears on their surfaces. What is so interesting about this is that much of the considerable list of benefits that weight lifting causes come directly from the damage that it causes to muscle fiber. Of course, the energy used in the original exercise increases circulation and burns fat, good things that you want to happen. However, both the increased circulation and fat-burning continue as the body starts to repair microdamage caused by the exercise. This is just the start of the good things that happen as the body's repair project continues. For instance, there is an enormously beneficial effect on hormone balance. In particular, an intense workout stimulates the pituitary gland to release human growth hormone. Not only does this extremely powerful hormone cause muscles to grow back stronger than they were, but it does this by very efficiently burning fat. The result is that you are replacing fat with muscle, or as the sports physiologists like to put it, you are increasing lean body mass. Let's take a brief overall look at what weight training does for you.

Strong, toned muscles are more metabolically active. By burning fat and increasing lean body mass you actually reset your metabolism to a higher rate. The result is that you end up burning more fat even when you are at rest. Strong, toned muscles also mean a healthier life and a shaped body that help you feel good about yourself. You will find that you are able to perform at a higher level of intensity in your favorite sports. Weight training stimulates bone cells to produce more bone. Studies have proven that it helps prevent the onset of late-life osteoporosis. Of course, weight training is preventive against late-life muscle loss as well, and people of all ages experience improved quality of life when the insulin/blood sugar balance is better controlled, oxygen capacity in-

creased, HDL cholesterol increased while LDL cholesterol is decreased, and blood pressure brought down—all things that happen in weight training.

Maybe it's because of improved circulation and hormone balance, maybe it's just because you can move with more confidence—whatever the reasons, soon after you start weight training, you will find yourself experiencing better moods along with the toned muscles. This is one reason why being a fitness trainer now has to be one of the greatest jobs in the world. More and more people come to my gym for the first time not really expecting the dramatic changes that take place as they follow their programs, and I have the great fun of being able to watch their surprise and delight. I can only add that I have seen the programs in this book work with just about anyone, young or old, as long as they made a commitment to do the exercises.

Being committed to your fitness program is important. Weight training will provide you with some strong inducements to sticking with it. First of all, there is the fact that most people see results from their efforts in a relatively short time. Then, there is what I call the gym effect. When they invented the gymnasium the ancient Greeks understood the wisdom of exercising the physical body in public, just as they understood the importance of exercising the mind in public, going to the *agora* to invent democracy. When you go to a gym the people you meet will provide the latest information and advice on exercise and nutrition. Their presence also generates an energy that picks you up on down days. The variety of equipment at a modern gym is an essential advantage—the ability to do both aerobic and anaerobic exercises in one place is one example of this advantage. Another is that when you have the right equipment available, you will never have a problem achieving enough intensity to produce training effect. You can get fit working out on your own, but it is a lot easier and a lot more fun to do it with friends.

I can give you tools in the form of knowledge that you need to get results, the tools you need to achieve the healthy, well-shaped body you have always wanted. I can tell you about the latest discoveries in nutrition and in the physiology of exercise. This book provides detailed programs that have been through such severe testing by trial and error that at this point the programs have worked many times successfully. If you can pay attention to the technical information and put in the sweat, you are all but guaranteed success.

You do provide another important element to the program. How well have you connected your mind to your body? I can tell you that I think of the body and mind as connected in a loop with information going both ways in pretty much equal intensity. To me, this is common sense. You tell your body what you want it to do, but you also listen carefully for signs from your body that tell you what it is capable of doing. I am sorry to say that one thing I have learned in the years I have spent working with people to help them be healthy and fit is that they cannot be depended on to have common sense. A lot of the people who come to train at gyms have to be told not to overdo it. It seems like the most frequent problem is that they see the mind-body loop as almost a one-way street, the overwhelming proportion of information going as orders from mind to body. The orders are overfamiliar—get thin, get strong, get perfect are representative examples of what I am talking about. The problem is, of course, that so much fierce energy goes into sending these messages, little information gets back from the body.

It is surprising sometimes to see how long this internal bullying can go on before trouble arises, but whether the time that passes is short or long, in the end trouble does inevitably arise. The problem needs to be put in context.

Let's face it: when people are listening exclusively to the body side of the mind-body loop they are getting very different advice, more like "You look good the way you are, everything is fine" (don't worry about tomorrow) and "Why don't we lie down and take a nice nap?" (ever notice how contented and guilt-free pets are about napping?). The body's normal urges do not lead to the gym.

However, you are a person who wants to look good and feel better, and you are willing to show up at the gym to do something to make this happen. There are definitely ways you can make the mind-body loop work for you, not against you. To understand one of them, we have to go back to expand our description of just what weight training is. You know that when the body repairs the muscle microdamage caused by exercise, the repaired muscle comes back stronger. The fact is this that this reaction to stress is only one of a whole series of such reactions that result in the body adapting to increased demands. Furthermore, this process of adaptation is progressive. What this means is that to a very great extent, the more you ask from your body, the more you get. The sports physiologists' term for this phenomenon is *training effect*.

The benefits I mentioned earlier—the stepped-up metabolism that uses more calories, improved muscle tone, increase in strength, stimulation of bone replacement, stimulation of hormonal response—all of these come from stressing the body long enough to coax it into adapting to a new level of performance. Training effect works on the principle of progressive overload; its intensity is built-in. Weight training uses controlled stress to get results.

When the training effect is in operation, you have nature working for you. This is the time to step back in your mind and just concentrate on the effects the exercise is having on your body. Nature provides us with keenly sensitive means to carry on this surveillance. Within the sensory nervous system, there is a specialized network of receptors, differentiated between muscles and tendons, that reports on all movement and muscle activity. Called proprioceptors, these nerve endings are the athlete's and the weight trainer's best friends. Developing your skill in using them will guarantee that you reach your goals in weight training.

Whatever those goals are—whether you want to sharpen your performance in your favorite sport, change something about your appearance that bothers you, or just feel stronger and more balanced as you go about your day-to-day activities—the weight training programs in this book can get you there. They give you that extra edge in life I call the Winning Factor.

Chapter Two

Nutrition

The Winning Factor can be looked at as a fabric woven from three strands: *food*, *exercise*, and *rest*. The three strands are equally important; all three must have your deliberate attention in order to make the program work. Let's begin by looking at diet first.

Too often, people tend to take the easy way out when it comes to diet. First, they think it doesn't matter all that much what they eat. Then, when they see that it does matter, they decide that all they have to do is eat one food, or avoid another one together, or even just take a pill to solve the problem. Since we have been taught to think of a weight problem as a medical problem, and since medical research tends to look for the "magic bullet" cure when it can, it's really not all that difficult to see how the search for easy answers got started. Nonetheless, remember that there are no magic bullets for weight control. The people who sell them are selling illusion.

Weight control is not what we intend to focus on here. What we are interested in is eating to be fit: not eating to live, but eating to be more alive. It makes sense to look at why you are eating. If you are doing it just to maintain life, or for pleasure, you can easily get into trouble with extra weight. However, when you eat to be fit, you are eating more the way that nature intended. Eating nature's way means learning the body's processes and patterns and working in conjunction with them when you make decisions about what is good or bad for you. It also means following the twin principles of moderation and balance. And it means that the diet program you follow is designed for your specific individual needs. Some effort has to go into learning how to eat this way, but once learned, it is not difficult to do. It certainly never requires the unnaturally extreme efforts of willpower that starvation diets can require.

When you take on an exercise routine, you are putting a direct wake-up call into your metabolism. Training sessions will stepup the entire metabolic cycle—increasing your heart beat, blood circulation, body heat, oxygen load, absorption of nutrients, then continuing the work through a clean-up removal of heat, carbon dioxide, minerals, and protein. If you supply your body with the kinds of food it needs to keep this metabolic process going strong while you exercise, it will not be long before you notice your stores of fat being replaced by lean muscle mass. You will be on your way to joining the ranks of people who forgot what it was like ever to have had a weight problem.

Use 5 Meal Plan:

King = Breakfast

Midmorning Snack

Prince = (Moderate) Lunch

Midafternoon Snack

Pauper = (Sparse) Dinner

TABLE 2-1

Body Fat Percentages				
Body Fat Rating	Excellent	Good	Fair	Poor
Women	15%	20%	25%	30%
Men	12%	18%	23%	28%
Deduct from Base	0%	–5%	–10%	–15%

TABLE 2-2

Daily Activity Expenditures Ratings		
Level	Lifestyle	Percent
Low	Sedentary, non-active	add 22%
Medium	Exercise one or two times a week, only slightly active	add 28%
High	Exercise three to four times a week, average active	add34%
Very High	Exercise five to seven times a week, plus sports activity, very active	add 40%

Now let's outline your personal nutrition guidelines. The first step is to make an estimate of the number of calories you would burn over a twenty-four-hour period if your metabolism remained at basal—that is, resting—rate for that long a time. The following formula does the estimate. If you are a man, use your weight in kilograms and multiply this figure times twenty-four. For a woman, the formula is slightly different to allow for the fact that women in general hold a little more body fat than men. Women simply multiply their weight in kilograms times .9 before multiplying it by twenty-four. Here are two examples, first a man weighing two hundred pounds:

$$\frac{200 \text{ lb.}}{2.2046 \text{ kg.}} = 90 \text{ kg.} \times 24 = 2{,}160 \text{ base calories}$$

Then for a woman weighing a hundred and twenty pounds:

$$.9 \times 120 \text{ lb.} = \frac{108 \text{ lb.}}{2.2046 \text{ kg.}} = 48 \text{ kg.} \times 24 =$$

$$1{,}152 \text{ base calories}$$

Whenever there is a radical change in your weight, this base figure can be recalculated to bring it up to date.

Before you begin making choices in nutrition, your base figure needs two adjustments. The first is subtraction and represents your ambitions for how thin you want to be. Table 2-1 gives a range of body fat percentages for men and women. After you place yourself in the chart according to how you evaluate your current condition, look to the bottom line of the chart to find the percentage of calories you are to deduct from your base calories.

TABLE 2-3

Breaking Down Your Total Calories

Activity	Protein	Carbohydrates	Fats
Losing fat while maintaining lean muscle mass	30%	50%	20%
Intense aerobic activities	25%	50%	25%
Heavy weight training at least four times a week	40%	40%	20%

Now let's return to our examples: Our man ranks himself as fair so he deducts 10 percent. That is 216 from 2,160 = a body-fat adjusted base of 1,944 calories.

Our woman ranks herself as fair as well and does the same: 115 from 1,152 equals a body-fat adjusted base of 1,036 calories.

The next adjustment you have to make is to add the calories to your base number that you need for the level of activities you have planned for yourself. Table 2-2 provides a chart of activity levels with the percentage of calories to add: This chart gives you the flexibility to adjust your calories to your activities on a daily basis.

The base figure you are using now has been tailored to you in three different ways: first by your body weight, second by your goals for the body fat percentage you want to reach, and third by the level of your activities.

Table 2-3 suggests how to break down your total calories for the day by percentages of protein, carbohydrate, and fat.

Balance these nutrients over five or six small meals, one every two or three hours, and be sure to consume some protein at each meal. On days when you train, zig-zag the protein and carbohydrate balances so that you eat carbohydrate-rich meals before the workout to store energy, and consume protein-rich meals after the workout for recovery. Conveniently packaged protein supplements, discussed in the next chapter, will help you keep to your schedule. The recipes and menus that follow are also designed to make it easier for you to make healthy food choices.

Try to combine careful management of your diet with some loose everyday guidelines, such as choosing complex carbohydrates like leafy green vegetables or potatoes more often than refined carbohydrates that contain too much sugar, or emphasizing unsaturated vegetable fats over saturated animal fats, or avoiding alcoholic beverages. In general, it is important to remember that you are the final judge of how any particular stage of the program is working for you.

> Empty Calories that have no nutritional value should be cut:
>
> Alcohol • Beer • Sugar

Finally, don't forget to drink lots of water. Water is the most important nutrient in your body, making up 70 to 75 percent of total body weight. It transports the other nutrients and carries waste material out. When fat is burned, waste products called ketone bodies are produced. Ketone bodies are processed by the kidneys and have to be removed quickly. Similarly, when protein is burned, nitrogen is produced and removed by the kidneys. These examples show how vital it is to drink enough water to flush away the waste products of our body's burned fuel. It is particularly important to remember to drink plenty of water when you are working out. Drink at least eight glasses a day.

Following are some working definitions of other key nutrients.

Carbohydrates

These substances are converted by the body into glycogen, stored in the muscle and used for energy. There are two types of carbohydrates.

Simple Carbohydrates are the quickest to be absorbed and include the following items: cakes, candies, cookies, corn syrup, fruits, honey, jams, molasses, soda, and maple and cane sugar.

Complex Carbohydrates are absorbed more gradually and include: beans, breads, carrots, cereals, corn, crackers, nuts, pasta, peas, potatoes, squash, and rice.

Proteins

Proteins comprise the structure of virtually every organ in the body and are responsible for growth and tissue repair. Your body cannot store proteins, so it is important to consume the ten essential amino acids every day. The best way is to eat five to six small servings of protein daily in addition to consuming the ten essential amino acids that cannot be made by the body like the non-essential aminos. If you do not take in enough protein, the first place your body will steal it from is the muscles. It does this in order to repair organs and other tissues. There are two categories of protein.

Complete Proteins, such as poultry, meat, fish, and dairy products, contain all the essential amino acids. These are normally higher in calories and fat than incomplete proteins.

Incomplete Proteins are best represented by most vegetables and fruits. In order for incomplete proteins to be effective, you must consume two to three different varieties per serving to get all essential aminos. This type of protein is normally higher in complex carbohydrates and fiber than complete proteins.

Cholesterol/Saturated Fats

Cholesterol is a fatty-type substance necessary for good health. It is essential for forming some hor-mones and for the formation of bile, which aids in the digestion of fats. Cholesterol is derived from foods of animal origin. The total fat calorie intake should never exceed thirty percent. An excessive storage or build-up of cholesterol in the body can contribute to the development of heart disease. Some guidelines for controlling fat intake are:

1. Substitute chicken, turkey, fish, and veal for red meat.
2. If consuming red meats, use only the leanest cuts and eat in moderation.
3. Fresh and dried legumes, such as peas and beans, as well as soy bean curd, can be used in place of meats.
4. Limit egg yolks. Use egg substitutes and egg whites instead of whole eggs in recipes.
5. Use low- or non-fat yogurt in place of ice cream.
6. Eat cheese having five or fewer grams of fat per serving.
7. Non-dairy creamers that contain palm, co-conut, or hydrogenated vegetable oils should only be used in moderation.
8. Cut back on butter intake and substitute with powdered butter.
9. Avoid deep-fried foods.

Along with getting enough water when you exercise, make sure you are also getting enough food. Never forget how important this is. When you don't eat enough, you slow down your metabolism and cause your body to catabolize lean mass. When you eat many small meals, you prevent this loss of muscle and actually help the body increase its rate of metabolism, burning fat into energy. Following are two different examples of menus for the whole day to give you some idea of how to plan for many small meals. You could alternate these two plans from one day to the next over a week or two. Following the plans there are different menus for each meal of the day: breakfast, lunch, and dinner, plus snacks. By selecting from these menus, you can plan further variations for your many-small-meals diet.

Typical Seven-Day Food Intake for Fat Loss and Lean Mass Increase

Serving sizes of foods should be adjusted to each individual's lean mass and energy expenditures

Monday, Wednesday, and Friday

7:00 to 8:00 A.M.
1 cup oatmeal
1 egg white
1 slice lite bread
1 slice cantaloupe
(4 aminos)

10:00 to 10:30 A.M.
1 baked potato
1 slice cantaloupe

12:00 to 12:30 P.M.
1 chicken breast
½ cup rice
1 baked potato
(3 aminos)

2:30 to 3:00 P.M.
1 chicken breast
Orange (juice)

5:30 to 6:00 P.M.
½ cup pasta salad
Veggies
(4 aminos)

Tuesday, Thursday, and Saturday

7:00 to 8:00 A.M.
1 bowl bran cereal
1 slice cantaloupe
(4 aminos)

10:00 to 10:30 A.M.
1 slice lite bread
1 slice cantaloupe

12:00 to 12:30 P.M.
½ cup pasta
1 chicken breast
Salad
(3 aminos)

1:00 to 2:00 P.M.
½ cup rice
Broccoli

5:00 to 6:00 P.M.
2 chicken breasts
1 cup rice
Veggies
Salad
(4 aminos)

Sunday

7:00 to 8:00 A.M.
1 cup oatmeal
1 slice lite bread
1 slice cantaloupe
(4 aminos)

12:00 to 12:30 A.M.
1 chicken breast
½ cup rice
(3 aminos)

5:00 to 6:00 P.M.
½ cup pasta
Salad
1 baked potato
Veggies
(4 aminos)

Nutrition Menu Plans for Increasing Metabolism

Select one of the following new suggestions for each meal.

Breakfast

- 8 oz. fruit juice, 2 egg whites with 1 yolk, 2 slices low-cal toast, 2 tbsp. spreadable fruit
- Low- or non-fat cereal, ½ cup skim milk, 1 cup fresh fruit, 1 cup fruit juice
- 1 whole wheat English muffin, ½ fresh melon, 2 egg whites with 1 yolk, 1 cup skim milk
- ½ cup cooked oatmeal, 2 tbsp. raisins, 2 cups skim milk, 1 cup fresh fruit
- 1 bran muffin, ½ fresh melon, 2 egg whites with 1 yolk, 1 cup skim milk
- 1 bagel, 1 tbsp. low-fat cream cheese, 1 cup fresh fruit, 1 cup skim milk

Lunch

- 2 slices of turkey breast, 2 slices whole wheat bread, 1 tbsp. mustard, lettuce, tomato, 1 piece of fruit
- ¾ cup chunk chicken, 1 tbsp. low-fat mayonnaise, ½ whole wheat pita, lettuce, tomato, 1 piece of fruit
- ¼ lb. broiled turkey burger or lean hamburger, low-cal roll, sliced onion, lettuce, and tomato, 1 tbsp. mustard or low-calorie ketchup, 1 piece of fruit
- ½ can tuna in water, 1 tbsp. low-fat mayonnaise, 2 slices whole wheat toast, slice of onion, 2 stalks of celery, 1 piece of fruit
- ¾ cup chunk chicken, 2 cups cooked pasta, ¼ cup low-fat Italian dressing, lettuce and tomato salad, lemon, 1 piece of fruit
- ¼ lb. broiled turkey or lean hamburger, 2 soft tortillas, shredded lettuce, tomato, and onion, 1 tbsp. mild salsa, 1 piece of fruit

Dinner

- ¼ lb. broiled tenderloin marinated in ¼ cup Worcestershire sauce, 1 baked potato, 1 tsp. plain low-fat yogurt, 4 broccoli spears
- Broiled chicken breast marinated in ¼ cup low-fat salad dressing, 1 cup cooked pasta, ½ cup French green beans
- ¼ lb. flounder with lemon and herbs, 1 cup red potatoes with garlic, ½ cup peas with onions, lettuce salad with cucumber and tomato
- 2 cups broiled scallops, 1 cup long-grain wild rice, ½ cup steamed pea pods, cucumber and tomato salad
- Grilled beef kabob, 6 cherry tomatoes, 3 halved fresh mushrooms, 3 halved small onions, sliced green pepper, 1 cup long-grain wild rice, spinach salad with egg white, garlic, lemon juice, and vinegar dressing
- 1½ cups cooked pasta, ½ cup each of carrots, broccoli, and cauliflower, ¼ cup fat-free Italian dressing, 2 tbsp. Parmesan cheese, 2 slices low-cal Italian bread

Snacks

You may have one of the following per day; your snack may be split between two meals if you prefer.

- 1 piece fruit or 1 cup of berries or grapes
- 3 cups oil-popped or 6 cups air-popped popcorn
- 6 rice cakes with spreadable fruit
- 1 cup fat-free yogurt with ½ cup diced fruit

Here are a few recipes that show how healthy meals can also be convenient to prepare.

Baked Italian Chicken

Coat chicken in low- or non-fat Italian dressing.
Bake at 350° for 45 minutes.
May also be broiled.

Turkey Stuffed Peppers

6 large peppers
3 lbs. ground turkey
1 cup cooked rice
1 cup whole wheat bread crumbs
2 tbsp. mustard
2 tbsp. parsley
1 medium onion, chopped
16 oz. low-sodium tomato sauce
6 slices low-fat, low-sodium cheese

Boil peppers for five minutes and drain. Combine turkey, rice, bread crumbs, mustard, onions, and parsley. Stuff mixture into peppers. Use remaining stuffing to make meatballs. Place peppers in baking dish and pour tomato sauce over top. Bake at 350° for two hours. Five minutes prior to removing peppers from oven, place cheese over the top of each pepper. Cheese is optional.

Roasted Chicken and Vegetables

1 large roasting bag
4 chicken breast halves
4 carrots cut in 2" lengths
6 celery stalks cut in 2" lengths
4 medium potatoes, quartered
3 medium onions, quartered
1 tsp. basil
1 tsp. thyme
4 tbsp. flour
¼ cup black pepper

Combine basil, thyme, flour, pepper, and water in roasting bag. Add chicken breasts and shake to coat. Add vegetables and coat. Arrange food in bag so vegetables are on bottom and the breasts are on top. Twist the end of bag to close and tie. Bake at 350° for one hour.

Baked Orange Roughy

2 orange roughy filets
Black pepper to taste
Paprika
Powdered butter substitute
2 tsp. lemon juice

Place orange roughy in glass baking dish, sprinkle seasoning over top. Bake at 350° for 35 to 45 minutes.

Turkey Burgers

1 lb. ground turkey breast
1 tbsp. ground parsley
¼ tsp. garlic powder
1 tbsp. black pepper
1 small onion, chopped
1 tbsp. Worcestershire sauce

Mix all ingredients together well and form into patties (4–6 depending on size desired). Broil in oven, grill, or fry in non-stick pan. Place on top of whole-grain bun and top with different vegetables.

Angel Hair Pasta with Turkey Pasta Sauce

1 package angel hair pasta
1 qt. low-sodium, low-calorie pasta sauce
1 lb. ground turkey breast
1 medium onion, chopped
1 large green pepper, chopped
4–6 sliced mushrooms (fresh)
1–2 cloves of garlic, chopped

Prepare pasta as directed on package. Mix onion, pepper, garlic, mushrooms, and turkey together. Brown in pan. Add to sauce and blend. Pour over pasta.

Tuna Variations

Baked potato topped with tuna and low-fat dressing
Baked potato topped with tuna, mixed with mustard
Tuna mixed with non-fat yogurt and seasoned with oregano on whole-grain bread.
   Mixture also can be stuffed into a tomato or green pepper
Mix diced apples with tuna and low-fat salad dressing

Cucumber Salad

1 large cucumber, sliced
½ cup onion, finely chopped
¼ cup non-fat yogurt
3–4 packages substitute sweetener to taste
⅛ tsp. black pepper

Mix all ingredients. Chill for several hours before serving.

Low-Cal Citrus Dressing

¼ cup lemon juice
3 tbsp. orange juice
3 tbsp. vegetable oil
3 packages substitute sweetener to taste
¼ tsp. celery seed

Place all ingredients in a bottle and shake. Refrigerate before serving.

Seasoned Potatoes

4–6 medium potatoes
¼ cup non-fat Italian dressing
Black pepper to taste

Cut potatoes, with skin on, into quarters. Brush potatoes with dressing and sprinkle pepper over top. Bake at 375° for 45 minutes.

Microwave Directions: Cook on high 4–6 minutes.

Steamed Apples

Peel apples, place in steamer for 4 minutes.
Remove, sprinkle with cinnamon or nutmeg.

Oat Bran Muffins

2½ cups oat bran cereal
2 tsp. brown sugar substitute
½ cup raisins
½ tbsp. baking powder
½ tsp. light salt
1 cup skim milk
4 oz. egg whites or egg substitute
1 tbsp. vegetable oil

Spray inside of muffin cups and place in muffin pan. Mix dry ingredients together. Mix oil, egg whites, and milk. Blend all ingredients and fill cups ⅔ full. Bake at 425° for 17 minutes or until brown.

Angel-Berry Cake

1 package angel food cake mix
1 lb. package frozen, unsweetened strawberries
  (thawed and drained)
1 small container of non-dairy whipped cream.

Prepare cake as directed on package and cool. Slice in half horizontally. Mix whipped cream and drained strawberries and spread bottom layer with ⅓ of mixture. Put cake top on and ice top and sides of cake with remaining mixture. Keep refrigerated.

High Protein Shake Variations

All these protein shakes should be mixed well and chilled.

- 1 pint whole milk
- 2 scoops natural ice cream
- 1 whole banana or ½ cup evaporated milk
- 4 tbsp. milk or egg protein

- 1 pint whole milk
- ½ cup evaporated milk
- 1 tbsp. peanut butter
- 1 tbsp. wheat germ

- 1 pint skim milk
- 1 cup milk protein powder
- ½ cup low-fat yogurt
- ½ cup sliced bananas or strawberries

- 1 pint of whole milk
- 1 tbsp. honey
- 1 banana

- ½ cup 1% or 2% milk
- ½ cup coconut milk
- ½ cup pineapple chunks
- 4 tbsp milk or egg protein

- 1 pint whole milk
- 3 oz. yogurt
- 6–8 strawberries
- 1 tbsp. honey

Nutritional Food Sources

The vitamins and minerals below are followed by the food sources that are highest in their quantities.

High Calcium Foods

These are important for healthy teeth and bones and are essential for normal blood clotting and functioning of muscles, nerves, and cell tissues. If your diet does not have enough calcium, it will be released from your bones.

Milk	Collard greens
Oysters	Salmon
Almonds	Sardines
Brewer's yeast	Spinach
Broccoli	Yogurt
Cottage cheese	Soybean curd

High Iron Foods

You need high iron foods for the formation of hemoglobin, which carries oxygen in the blood. They also increase resistance to stress and disease.

Lima beans	Molasses
Lean beef	Liver
Brewer's yeast	Eggplant
Breads	Pasta
Broccoli	Potatoes
Carrots	Rice
Oatmeal	Chicken
Mushrooms	Creamed wheat cereal
Apricots	

High Potassium Foods

Proper functioning of all muscle contractions and metabolism of carbohydrates and proteins depend on high-protein foods. Along with sodium, they regulate the amount of water in the individual cells.

Raw tomatoes	Clams
Tuna	Milk
Chicken	Flounder
Bananas	Avocados
Potatoes	Spinach
Brussels sprouts	Yogurt
Lima beans	Orange juice

High Magnesium Foods

These aid in releasing energy from foods that are consumed.

Almonds	Bran
Apples	Soybean curd
Peanuts	Shrimp
Pecans	Cheese
Pistachios	Lima beans
Hazelnuts	Whole-grain cereals
Spinach	

High Vitamin A Foods

You need vitamin A for proper growth of hair, teeth, eyes, and bones. It also helps the immune system.

Milk (whole)	Pumpkin
Peas	Apricots
Yams	Green beans
Cantaloupe	Asparagus
Broccoli	Peaches
Carrots	

High Vitamin C Foods

These aid in the absorption of iron and are needed for collagen production and healthy gums.

Brussels sprouts	Cantaloupe
Broccoli	Green peppers
Parsley	Cauliflower

High Vitamin D Foods

Calcium and phosphate metabolism are regulated with the help of vitamin D.

Salmon	Eggs
Milk	Herring
Sardines	Liver

High Vitamin E Foods

These protect cells and membranes from wear and tear.

Cod liver oil	Peanuts
Corn oil	Pecans
Olive oil	Almonds
Sesame oil	Walnuts
Soybean oil	Wheat germ oil
Sunflower oil	

High Vitamin B_1 Foods and Foods with Thiamin

Vitamin B_1 and thiamin aid in breaking down carbohydrates into glucose

Asparagus	Rice
Cereal	Veal
Liver	Oysters
Dried beans	Milk (2%)
Lima beans	Orange juice
Pasta	Lamb

Niacin and Vitamin B_3 Foods

These provide energy to the cells for proper growth.

Asparagus	Veal
Lean beef	Yogurt
Brussels sprouts	Liver
Broccoli	Hamburger
Chicken	Cottage cheese
Eggs	Milk
Tuna	

Riboflavin and Vitamin B_2 Foods

These help to break down proteins, carbohydrates, and fats into energy.

Asparagus	Whole-grain cereal
Raw apples	Pecans
Bran	Hazelnuts
Avocados	Almonds
Lima beans	Spinach
Wheat germ	Soybean curd
Cheese	Cashews

Pyridoxine and Vitamin B_6 Foods

Vitamin B_6 and pyroxidine aid in metabolizing amino acids.

Bananas	Milk
Veal	Fish
Cabbage	Liver
Oatmeal	Beef
Potatoes	

Cobalamin and Vitamin B_{12} Foods

These are important in the development of red blood cells.

Beef	Eggs
Liver	Fatty fish
Veal	Cheese
Lamb	Milk
Chicken	

Cobalamin and Vitamin K Foods

These are important for proper blood clotting.

Asparagus	Liver
Broccoli	Spinach
Cabbage	Turnip greens
Cheese	Whole wheat bread
Lettuce	

Water

Water is the most important nutrient of all! Most fruits are 75 percent water by weight. Skim milk is at least 91 percent water.

Watermelon   Oranges
Cucumbers   Raw oysters
Lettuce   Skim milk
Raw tomatoes Cooked pasta
Celery

Nutritional Maintenance

Foods to Use

Poultry: Turkey, chicken, skinless white meat.
Fish and seafood: Tuna in water, flounder, haddock, pollack, scallops, and shrimp.
Lean beef
Egg whites or egg substitutes
Non-fat dairy products
Oatmeal
Rice/rice cakes
Baked potatoes
Unrefined grains
Whole-grain breads
Cereals
Fresh salad
Green vegetables
Fresh fruits and juices
Low-fat melba toast
Low-calorie preserves
Low-calorie salad dressing
Herbs and spices
Light salt and sugar substitute
Vinegar
Mustard and light ketchup
Low-calorie drinks (in moderation)

Foods to Avoid

Pork and bacon
Canned meats and vegetables
Cooking and salad oils
Seeds and nuts
Coconut
Avocados
Corn
Butter
Lard
Sugar
Salt
Gravies and sauces
Whole dairy products
Corn starch
Egg yolks
Refined grains
Pastries
Filler meats: bologna, sausages, hot dogs and scrapple.

Many of my clients lead very busy lives and have to follow schedules that make it difficult to maintain high standards in their diets. This is particularly a problem for people who have to travel a lot and end up eating at fast food restaurants. Table 2-4 is a list of suggestions that I have developed over the years to help anyone who has this problem.

TABLE 2-4

Tips for Eating on the Road and At Fast Food Restaurants

Breakfast

The Quickie
440 Calories • 21 gm. Fat
1 Fast Food Cinnamon Danish Pastry

vs. Healthy Choice
0 gm. Fat
2½ Fast Food Fat-Free Apple Bran Muffins

Sunny Side Up
445 Calories • 26 gm. Fat
1 Egg Fried in Butter
3 Strips Bacon
2 Slices White Toast
2 Pats of Butter
2 Tsps. Strawberry Jam

vs. Healthy Choice
16 gm. Fat
2 Eggs Fried in Non-Stick Non-Fat Vegetable
   Spray
1½ English Muffins
1 Pat of Butter
1 Fresh Orange

In the Box
600 Calories • 23 gm. Fat
1 cup Granola Style Cereal
2⅓ cup Whole Milk

vs. Healthy Choice
8 gm. Fat
2¾ cup Unsweetened Whole Wheat Cereal
1¾ cup 1% Milk
1 Banana

In the Toaster
210 Calories • 6 gm. Fat
1 Blueberry Toaster Pastry
Danish Pastry

vs. Healthy Choice
3 gm. Fat
3 Slices Whole Wheat Toast
2 Tsp. Sugar-Free Blueberry Preserves

On the Side
110 Calories • 9 gm. Fat
3 Medium Slices of Bacon (2.4 oz)

vs. Healthy Choice
5 gm. Fat
2½ Slices of Canadian Bacon

Coffee Break
235 Calories • 13 gm. Fat
1 Glazed Donut

vs. Healthy Choice
6 gm. Fat
1 Small Blueberry Muffin
1 Banana

Lunch

Drive-Thru Sandwich
600 Calories • 34 gm. Fat
1 Fast Food Double Cheeseburger with Double
   Decker Bun

vs. Healthy Choice
16 gm. Fat
2 Fast Food Grilled Chicken Fillet Sandwiches

Sandwich
320 Calories • 17 gm. Fat
1 Frozen Ham & Cheese Croissant
⅔ cup Whole Milk

vs. Healthy Choice
6 gm. Fat
Bagel with One Slice of Lean Ham

Fast Food Seafood
200 Calories • 11 gm. Fat
3 oz. Batter Dipped Fried Fish

vs. Healthy Choice
3 gm. Fat
6 oz. Baked or Grilled Sole

Chickening Out

350 Calories • 18 gm. Fat
6 Fast-Food Deep Fried Nuggets w/Sweet and Sour Dipping Sauce

vs. Healthy Choice
11 gm. Fat
4½ Skinless Drumsticks, Roasted

Picnic Basket

330 Calories • 23 gm. Fat
1 Bologna Sandwich w/2 Slices Mixed Grain Bread & 1 Tbsp. Mayonnaise

vs. Healthy Choice
3 gm. Fat
2 Turkey Loaf Sandwiches on Mixed Grain Bread w/Lettuce, Tomato & Mustard

On the Side

21 gm. Fat
1 cup Potato Salad w/Regular Mayonnaise

vs. Healthy Choice
360 Calories • 12 gm. Fat
2 Ears of Corn
2 Pats of Butter

Afternoon Treat

13 gm. Fat
23 Chocolate Covered Peanuts

vs. Healthy Choice
2 gm. Fat
67 Seedless Grapes

Dinner

Salad

160 Calories • 14 gm. Fat
1 cup Iceberg Lettuce w/2 Tbsp. Italian Dressing

vs. Healthy Choice
7 gm. Fat
2 cups Iceberg Lettuce, 2½ oz. Packaged Croutons, ½ Tomato w/1 Tbsp. Low-Fat Vinaigrette Dressing

Soup

200 Calories • 14 gm. Fat
1 cup Canned Cream of Mushroom Soup

vs. Healthy Choice
6 gm. Fat
2½ cup Minestrone

Entree

230 Calories • 9 gm. Fat
4 oz. Chicken Breast w/Skin, Roasted

vs. Healthy Choice
8 gm. Fat
5 oz. Pork Tenderloin, Roasted

Pasta

520 Calories • 20 gm. Fat
2 cups Canned Spaghetti and Meatballs in Tomato Sauce

vs. Healthy Choice
6 gm. Fat
2¾ cups Canned Spaghetti in Tomato Sauce.

Vegetables

290 Calories • 10 gm. Fat
1 cup Potatoes Au Gratin from Mix

vs. Healthy Choice
6 gm. Fat
2½ Medium Baked Potatoes (no skin) w/1½ Tbsp. Non-Fat Yogurt & ½ Tbsp. Chopped Chives

Dessert

320 Calories • 10 gm. Fat
1 cup Chocolate Pudding Made w/Whole Milk.

vs. Healthy Choice
0 gm. Fat
2 cups Gelatin

Snacks

Movie Munchies

420 Calories • 35 gm. Fat
4 cups Oil-Popped Popcorn w/2 Tbsp. Butter Flavoring

vs. Healthy Choice
4 gm. Fat
13½ cups Air-Popped Salted Popcorn

TV Munchies
550 Calories • 38 gm. Fat
1 Bag Corn Chips (3 oz.) w/3 Tbsp. Avocado
   Dip

vs. Healthy Choice
14 gm. Fat
2 Whole Wheat Pitas
½ cup Hummus

Shirt-Pocket Treat
510 Calories • 24 gm. Fat
1 King-Sized Snickers Bar

vs. Healthy Choice
0 gm. Fat
64 Wild Cherry Life Savers

Taking a Dip
300 Calories • 22 gm. Fat
20 Potato Chips
4 Tbsp. Onion Dip

vs. Healthy Choice
0 gm. Fat
124 Carrot Sticks
½ cup Non-Fat Yogurt

The Cookie Jar
120 Calories • 6 gm. Fat
1 Packaged Chocolate Chunk Cookie

vs. Healthy Choice
2 gm. Fat
2 Packaged Fig Bars

From the Freezer
195 Calories • 7 gm. Fat
Ice-Cream Sandwich

vs. Healthy Choice
2 gm. Fat
3 Fruit Popsicles

TABLE 2-4

Fast Foods Lowest in Fat

Company Product	Percent of Fat Grams
Side Salad (Several Companies)	0
McDonald's apple bran muffin	0
McDonald's Wheaties	0
Long John Silver's green beans	0
TCBY Non-fat frozen yogurt	0
Wendy's three-bean salad	0
Arby's Old-fashioned chicken noodle soup	Less than 1
Long John Silver's light portion baked fish dinner	Less than 1
McDonald's low-fat milk shake	Less than 1
Dunkin Donuts plain bagel	Less than 1
KFC Mashed potatoes and gravy	Less than 1
Hardees pancakes (no margarine)	Less than 1
Long John Silver's Rice Pilaf	1
KFC corn on the cob	1
McDonald's chunky chicken salad	1
Wendy's chili	2
Wendy's seafood salad	2
McDonald's McLean deluxe	2

Fish or Chicken: Eat these baked or broiled (no sauces).
Burgers: Avoid "big"-sounding beef sandwiches. Regular hamburgers are better.
Roast Beef: It is easier to find low-fat roast beef than burgers.
Avoid sauces. Low-fat foods in restaurants are becoming increasingly available. Each of the foods on this chart contain two teaspoons of fat or less. Omitting tartar sauce or mayonnaise will further reduce the fat content of many other sandwiches as well.

Chapter Three

Supplements

I hope I have made it clear to you how important it is to support your exercise program with a diet that provides an optimum balance of protein, carbohydrates, and fat. Why, then, you might ask, is there another separate chapter on supplements for that diet? The answer is found in the word *exercise*. When you exercise regularly, especially when you exercise with definite goals in mind, it just makes sense to take any obvious step that will help you meet your goals.

The truth is that experience has taught us that supplements do work—they can help. Another reason to consider taking them is that there is such an intriguing array out there now to choose from. A whole army of brilliant scientific minds seems to be working night and day to come up with new discoveries. DHEA and co-enzyme Q-10 are just two discoveries that have received publicity in recent years.

Take the case of the old tried-and-true multimineral supplement. Recent research on biological transmutation by Prof. Louis C. Kervran has revolutionized the delivery of trace minerals to our bodies' cells. Manufacturing trace minerals in colloidal, anionic, or spray-dried form has greatly increased the effectiveness of these all-important nutrients for bones, muscles, and nerves.

We are truly living in the age of the super-supplements. They have gone from being simply insurance against possible deficiencies in the diet to being perceptible performance-enhancers in their own right. Look for companies that use the latest processes: colloidal minerals, custom enzyme blends, and negatively charged formulas.

However, always remember that as good as they are, supplements are never a reason for neglecting to eat a healthy, balanced diet. The truth is that supplements are only truly effective when combined with a proper diet.

This area is also one where it is a very good idea to be aware of your individual needs. Follow manufacturers' suggestions and then carefully evaluate any supplement you take for the effect it has on you. What I am offering you in the list that follows is a discussion of some of my favorite supplements, the ones that have worked well for me.

Protein Powder

As we explained in the first chapter, the Winning Factor takes you to higher levels of activity in your life. This means that you will have to increase your intake of protein proportionately. As you take control of your diet, you will quickly discover that protein foods are a little more difficult to deal with than carbohydrates. They take longer to prepare before you can eat them and longer to digest afterward, so that fitting them into a busy schedule can become a chore. Therefore, the availability of well-made isolated protein powders is a real blessing for the exercise enthusiast. Carefully processed from healthful sources (I prefer whey- or egg-based formulas), they are an indispensable item for your supplement menu. I take protein powder in a shake fifteen minutes after training. This provides protein for the body to repair stress and damage brought on by the workout. If this isn't done, the repair process, a stage of metabolism called catabolism, will take too much protein from your lean muscle mass.

Those who take protein supplements need a reminder about the importance of moderation in the way diet fits into the individual program. In this case, you want to be careful to adjust the amount of protein you eat to the intensity level of your workouts. Too much protein in a body that does not need it to repair bone, muscle, and tissue is a bad idea. If the process of digesting protein gets extended for too long, it can overstress the kidneys. Too much protein also has a dehydrating effect and in general robs the body of energy.

Amino Acids

These fundamental constituents of protein play an important role in metabolism. There are twenty-four of them, including an essential nine that must come from outside food sources: isoleucine, phenylalanine, histidine, leucine, threonine, lysine, tryptophan, methionine, and valine. Tablets that provide a selected range of all twenty-four are a useful way to supplement your protein needs. They prevent deficiencies as well as providing a protective base against imbalances that taking any further individual amino acids might cause.

Because they come in tablet form, amino supplements are very convenient to take. You should, however, make sure that the tablet or capsule you purchase provides the actual amino acids and not just more protein powder packaged into pill form. As with protein powder, adjust your intake to your activity level.

I take two or three tablets at mid-morning, mid-afternoon, and one hour before bedtime—this last dose on an empty stomach. Several amino acids listed below deserve to mentioned individually. I take these in a low-calorie carbohydrate drink immediately after training. Amino acids should not be taken with milk.

Creatine Monohydrate

This supplement is a formula that duplicates a naturally occurring metabolite of three amino acids, methionine, glycine, and arginine. It is designed to directly affect muscle cells, where, in phosphate form, it increases the cell's ability to store ATP, adenosine triphosphate, the source of energy used by the cells for muscle contraction. Research shows that creatine adds intensity to training and at the same time improves recovery. It is one of my favorite supplements.

OKG (Ornithine alphaketogutarate)

This amino acid is singled out from the others because of its particularly effective role in muscle tissue repair. It has been clinically shown to decrease muscle protein catabolism, improve nitrogen retention in muscle tissue, stabilize insulin levels in the bloodstream, and increase the speed of protein synthesis and muscle recovery. This is a supplement that has withstood the test of time.

L-Glutamine

This amino acid is used up rapidly during metabolic stress, partly because it combats a too-severe buildup of the steroid hormone cortisol and delays the onset of the muscle soreness that accompanies strenuous anaerobic exercise. Supplementing this amino has a strong anti-catabolic effect, it is great for recovery and muscle building, and at the same time it is even boosting your immune system. L-glutamine can be added to the broad-range tablet that you take at bedtime to stimulate the body's natural release of human growth hormone, a process that the pituitary gland triggers while we are sleeping.

Vitamins

The official line on vitamins is that you can get them in a well-balanced diet. Technically this is true, just as it is true that vitamins work in very small amounts (but most food sources are vitamin deficient, due to pesticides and depleted soil). The same things can be said about minerals and enzymes, which are also on this list of supplements. The reason I recommend all three of them, vitamins, minerals, and enzymes, is that I find from experience that taking them makes a difference. Actually, many studies done with athletes back up this use of vitamin and mineral supplements. The evidence is strong that they increase energy, especially when a body is asked to meet the sharp demands made by regular exercise.

A moderately high-potency formula is best, perhaps combined with the wide-range amino acid supplement recommended above. B vitamins are particularly important for metabolism of proteins; C and E are valuable antioxidants and also protect the health of blood vessels and cellular walls. Unless a doctor prescribes them for you, never take large amounts—so-called megadoses—of vitamins.

Colloidal Minerals

Minerals are essential building material for blood, nerve cells, muscle tissue, bones, and teeth. Though they only account for five percent of our body weight, the seventeen essential minerals, performing interrelated functions, are as important as any element in our diet. Plants absorb them easily from the ground so they are in pretty much all the food we eat. Why, then, are critical mineral deficiencies often found in large sections of the population? Stories about the health dangers from too little calcium or chromium are only the most recent examples of mineral deficiency scares.

The answer may be back in the ground where the plants are growing and in the methods of modern agriculture. Too often, the food available to us has been grown in depleted soil and in soil that for some time has been artificially enriched by chemicals. This fact is reason enough to consider taking a mineral supplement. Another reason to do so is that minerals are lost at an exorbitant rate when we exercise. To ward off fatigue, it is important that we replace them. When exercising regularly, magnesium, calcium, and potassium are particularly important.

As we mentioned earlier in this chapter, minerals are now available in a new form, colloidal suspension. If they have been processed this way, your body will absorb them much more efficiently, greatly increasing their effectiveness.

Enzymes

Enzymes are involved in a very broad range of the body's biochemical reactions. They are necessary for the very functioning of our metabolism, as well as for cleaning and repairing tissue. When people suffer enzyme deficiency, the symptoms can be serious, ranging from every aspect of digestive upset to overall fatigue and proneness to allergies. Unfortunately, since the enzymes produced by our bodies need to work with enzymes that come with our food, enzyme deficiencies are all too common.

The trouble comes from the fact that enzymes in food sources are unstable and easily inactivated by high temperatures or exposure to certain chemicals. The result is that the cooked and otherwise processed food we eat is not enzyme-active. Eating raw fruits and vegetables will help, but often not completely, because raw food requires more enzymes when it is being digested, and it is also often affected by processing by shippers and by the long period of time from harvesting to your consumption. All of this adds up to greatly reduced enzymatic effectiveness for much of the raw food available to us.

Since you want to focus on optimizing your metabolism, it makes sense to take an enzyme supplement. Look for a formula that includes the following individual enzymes: amylase, lactase, lipase, protease, and cellulase.

Co-Enzyme Q-10

This enzyme co-factor has to be present for the part of the metabolic process that produces ATP, which, as you remember from my description of creatine monohydrate, is a very important energy trigger in the muscles. A lot of ordinary life stress, including aging, lowers our body's ability to produce co-enzyme Q-10 on its own. The result is that people often find it has a dramatically good effect when taken as a supplement.

Besides boosting energy production, it also functions as an antioxidant. It has been used therapeutically to strengthen both blood circulation in the heart and the immune system. I have found that it fits very well into my training program.

DHEA

DHEA, produced by the adrenal glands, is the most prolific hormone in your body. As a pro-hormone, its most valuable function is to form the base from which many other key metabolites are derived. For this reason, when its production begins to fall off after you pass your early twenties, the effect on your body is systemic, the most notable being a falling off of metabolic efficiency and energy. We have found that supplementing it corrects the loss of energy and many other of the general effects of aging. For this reason, it is very useful in a training program, especially for people starting out in less than peak condition.

Balancing Nutrition

Sports nutrition is definitely a trial-and-error proposition, but it is not less important for that fact. The truth is that taking pains with it and paying attention to its effects leads to improved performance. If you try, you will be able to identify the foods that provide energy, strength, and endurance. Notice if something you take improves recovery or if it helps your body stand up to more intense workouts. Knowledgeable athletes constantly revise their eating strategies to find the combination of food and supplements that provides optimum strength and energy. Develop and use your own skills at monitoring your body's internal states to do the same thing.

Chapter Four

Stretching

You are convinced fitness is important, and you are ready to work to get in shape. The question is, how do you start? The answer is that every workout you do should start with a warm-up period and end with a cool-down period. These transition stages into and out of the main exercise can include any light activity that gets your circulation going, from walking to a very light form of the main exercise itself. The one thing your warm-up and cool-down should always include is a series of stretches.

High school gym class may have put most people off stretching exercises for life. In any case, they're not the glamorous part of exercise. They don't sculpt muscles or make them bigger; they don't put the big demands on your body that cause it to burn up stores of fat and carbohydrates. What many people don't realize, however, is that almost none of us are ready to start doing the glamorous exercises just like that. The reason for this is that our muscles adapt only too well to nature's economical way with energy. Their ordinary, everyday tasks of holding our bodies up against the force of gravity, say, or going through the limited actions involved in working at a desk are what they are always ready to do. Compared to the muscles you need for weight training or running, they are short, stiff, and undersupplied by our vascular systems with blood and lymph.

If you ask these shortened, closed-down muscles to suddenly do heavy work, their first reaction is

to shorten and close down a little more, as if they need to resist for a while to figure out what is going to happen. If you keep working against their resistance, they will eventually lengthen out and warm up. So what avoiding stretching has got you is a workout in which you spend extra energy fighting against nature. Experience has taught us that this is not the best way to work out. We stretch before we exercise, because if we don't, we find that at best we have a shorter, less pleasant session, and at worst we can end up with definitely unpleasant strain or sprain injuries. There's nothing glamorous about injuries either—they usually mean no exercise at all while you wait out the healing.

When you stretch muscles and tendons, their blood supply is immediately increased, literally warming them up. This in turn increases their elasticity and speeds up muscle contraction response time. Stretching is also very effective in promoting a better range of motion around your joints. You will find out later in the program when you are lifting weights that moving them through a full range of motion is necessary to fully stimulate the muscles you are working. A full range of motion with a stretching warm-up becomes a dangerous overextension without a warm-up.

There is another benefit provided by stretching that should be mentioned. While it provides a transition for your body from inaction to action, it also often takes your mind on a parallel transition, one from being distracted, even anxious, to being calm and securely centered. In this more intuitive state you can do a better job of monitoring your interior states, an important skill to work at when you exercise regularly.

Mention of this last benefit also leads to a warning. While stretching is absolutely essential for preventing injuries, this does not mean that you cannot be injured while you are stretching. A word here about the physiology of the muscles explains why. When you ask a muscle to act, it can only contract. This doesn't mean that it is incorrect to say that we stretch a muscle, it just means that it would be more explicit if we said that we stretch a muscle by asking another muscle opposing it to contract. Trouble arises when we ask for a stretch from a muscle that can't provide it. Pulled out as they are between tendon attachments to bone, in a position we have selected, stretched muscles are pretty much at our mercy. If these muscles decide that you are not showing them enough mercy, they will make you know it by doing the only thing they can do, suddenly trying to contract. This causes pain, sometimes lots of pain. It is not good for you. The catch phrase, "no pain, no gain," definitely does not apply to stretching. The wise thing to do is carefully monitor the muscle you are stretching. You will learn that there is a point near pain where the muscle is just thinking about contracting. When you gently push against this point in the exercises, you will find your muscle flexibility increasing from session to session. Just remember not to try to hurry or push beyond it. Other rules for stretching are:

- Never bounce or swing your body against the resistance of a stretch.
- Be very careful when testing injured muscles, and don't test them at all if they are still painful.
- Be careful when working known trouble spots.
- Go slowly, step by step, with controlled movements.
- Breathe in going into the stretch, breathe out slowly as you release it, and try to relax into a little deeper stretch.

Stretching exercises are an important part of your warm-up and cool-down routines, but you do not begin a warm-up with stretches. The first thing you do before serious exercise is at least five minutes of some light to moderate whole body activity like riding a stationary bicycle, walking a treadmill, or jogging easily around an indoor track. You can even just lie on your back and "bicycle" your legs in the air for a few minutes, as long as you do enough overall activity to raise your body's core temperature. This gives your lungs and heart a chance to respond gradually to the demands of exercise.

For example, as you do this part of the warm-up, your blood starts to thin and circulate more easily. Adjusting the blood flow in this way prevents the serious strain on your heart that can result if you begin strenuous working of the muscles with your blood cool and thickened. Light activity is the natural, unstressful way to get a workout going and is as important to do if you are experienced and conditioned as it is for the out-of-shape beginner. Once you have warmed the major muscle groups, doing some stretches will prepare you for the individual exercises.

Ten Basic Stretches

Following are ten basic stretches for you to use, and descriptions of the five types of stretching.

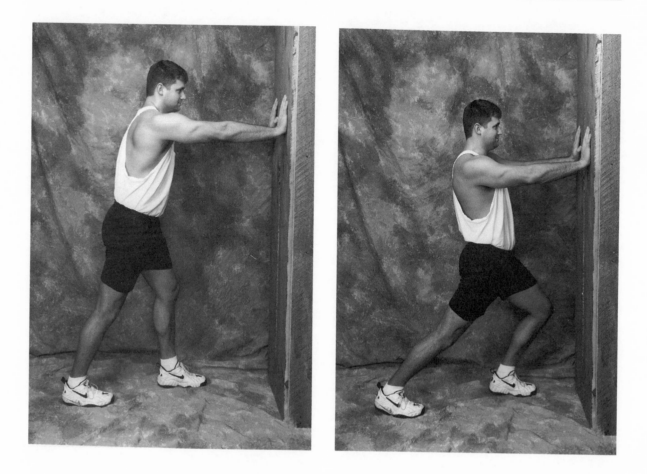

Ankle, Calf, and Achilles Tendon Stretches

Place both hands against a wall with arms straight at shoulder height. Move your right leg back a step, keeping your knee flexible and your heel on the floor. Step forward with your left leg, stretching the back of your right leg. Hold for ten seconds, then alternate legs.

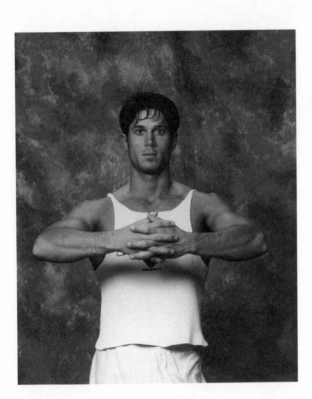 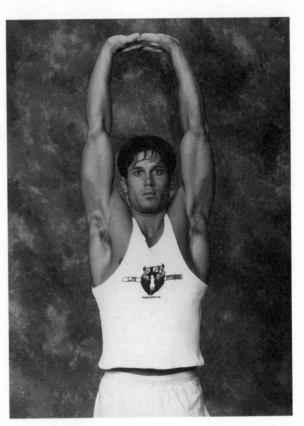

Arm and Shoulder Stretches

Lace your fingers together, then stretch and push your arms, elongating them overhead with palms toward ceiling. Hold for ten seconds.

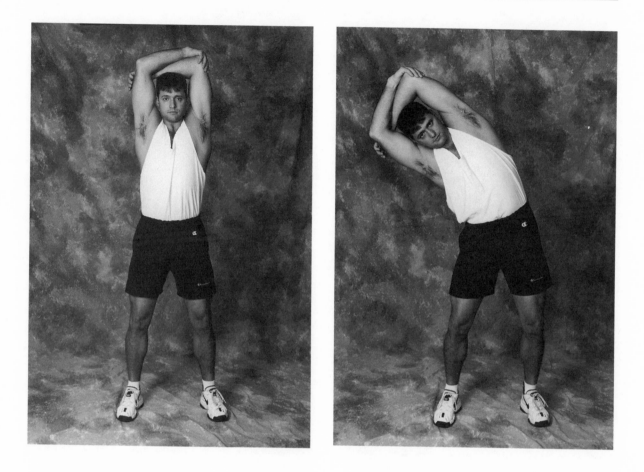

Side and Arm Stretches

Cross both arms over your head and grasp one elbow with the opposite hand. Gently pull the elbow behind your head and bend at the waist in the same direction, stretching muscles in the back of your arm, shoulder, and side. Knees should be slightly bent for balance. Repeat with the other arm. Hold for twenty seconds.

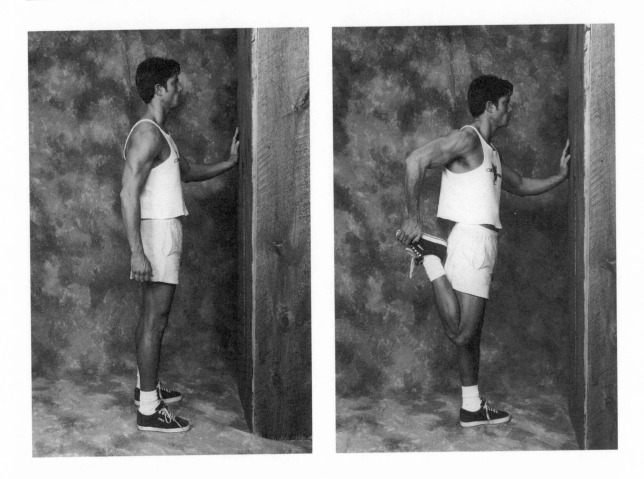

Quadriceps Stretches

If necessary for balance, place the right hand against a wall, then reach behind with the right hand and grasp the top of your right foot. Gently pull the heel up toward the gluteus. Hold for a count of ten. Repeat on the opposite side. This will stretch the entire quadriceps from knee to waist.

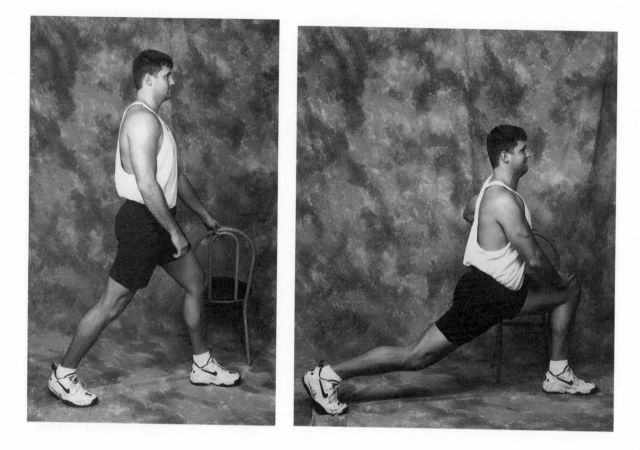

Hip and Groin Stretches

Take one giant step forward until the knee of your rear leg almost touches the floor. If necessary, rest your hands on the floor for stability. The front leg is bent with lower leg perpendicular to the foot. For a count of ten, push hips slowly toward the floor. Repeat on the opposite side.

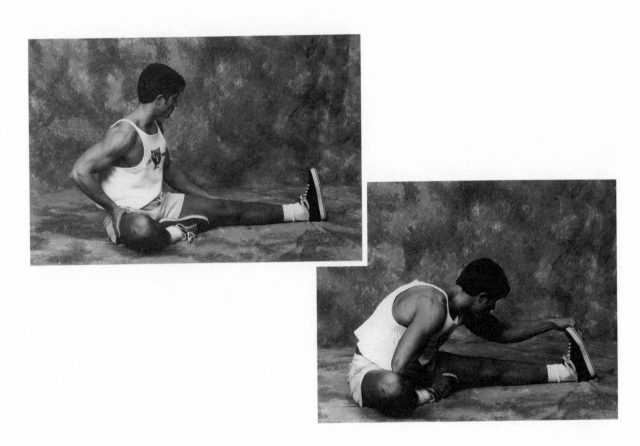

Hamstring and Lower Back Stretches

Sit on the floor with one leg outstretched slightly to the side. Place bottom of the opposite foot against the inner thigh of the outstretched leg. With the foot flexed toward the shin, slowly stretch down toward the foot of your outstretched leg. Hold for a count of ten, feeling the stretch at the back of your leg and in the lower back. Make sure you stretch both sides.

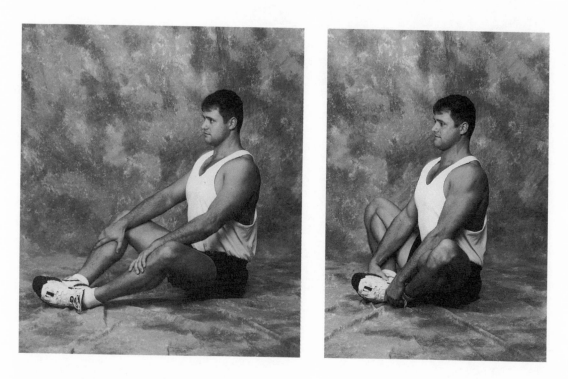

Inner Thigh and Groin Stretches

Sit on the floor and place the bottoms of your feet together. Pull your feet toward your groin. Placing your elbows against your lower legs, try gently pushing both knees toward the floor, feeling a good stretch for the inner muscles of the thighs.

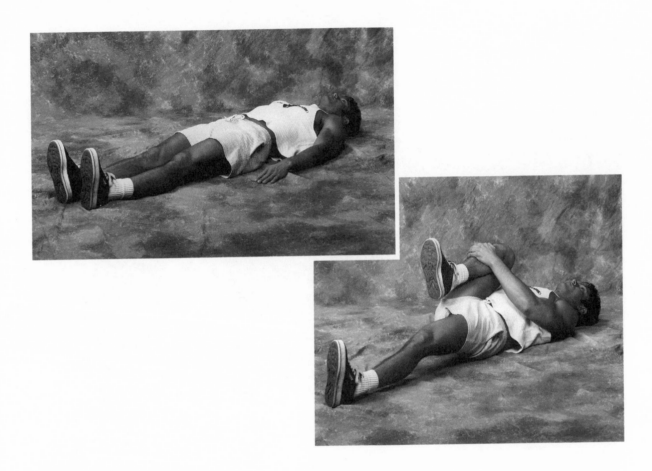

Buttock and Hamstring Stretches

Lie on your back with both legs straight. Pull one knee toward your chest, using both hands. Hold for ten seconds and repeat with the opposite leg.

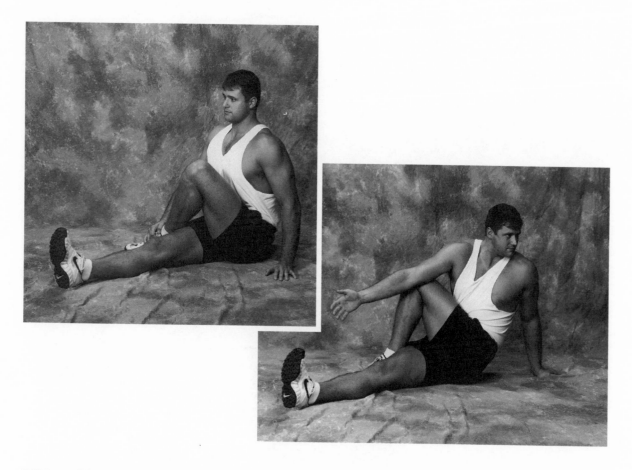

Mid and Lower Back Stretches

Sit on the floor with your right leg straight out. Cross your left foot over the outside of your right leg and place the foot down flat on the floor. Leaning to the left with the left hand on the floor for support, place the right elbow against the outer knee of the bent left leg. Stretch both sides equally.

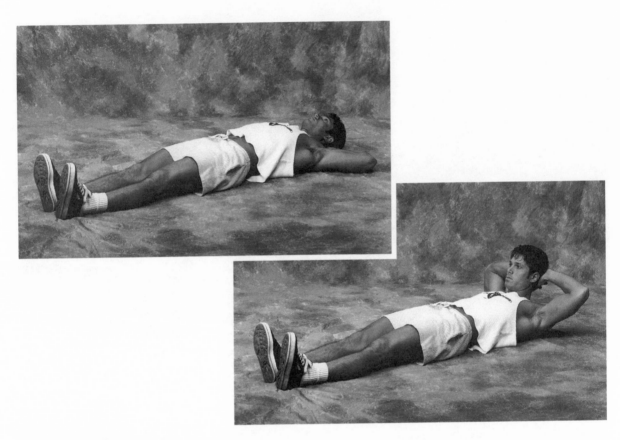

Neck Stretches

Lie on your back with both hands behind your head. Slowly pull your chin toward your chest, using your arms. Slowly return your head to the floor.

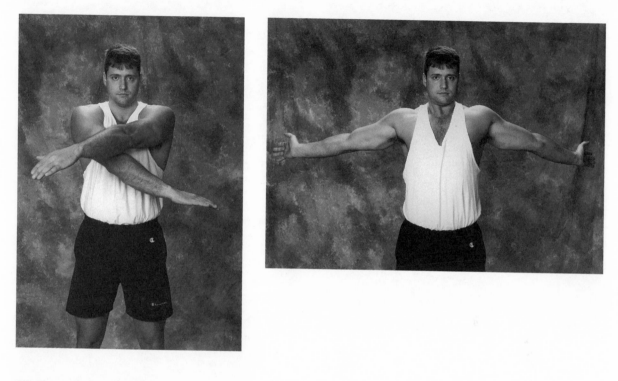

Dynamic Stretching

These stretches are used primarily by athletes who need to increase their range of motion for sports skills. Dynamic stretching involves swinging the arms and legs in a controlled manner. Various patterns can be utilized. When stretching dynamically, you must be careful not to exceed your present range of motion for the joint(s) being stretched, or injury could result. Two methods can be used to ensure the safety of this type of stretching:

- An even, controlled rhythm must be established, with swinging movements initially well within your range of motion. Gradually increase the amplitude of the movement until you are at the desired level of tension at the same time you come to the end-point of movement.

- During some stretches, particularly those for the legs, you can swing (kick) your leg into your hand, which stops the stretch at the end of each swing. Your nervous system will anticipate this, and as a result, the "stretch reflex" will be minimized or even eliminated. Please bear in mind that these are specialized movements and that care must be taken with their use.

> ### Types of Stretches
>
> There are five types of stretching: Dynamic, PNF, Isometric, Fascial, and Static. Dr. Frederick Carl Hatfield, Ph.D., of the I.S.S.A. gives an excellent description of the different types.

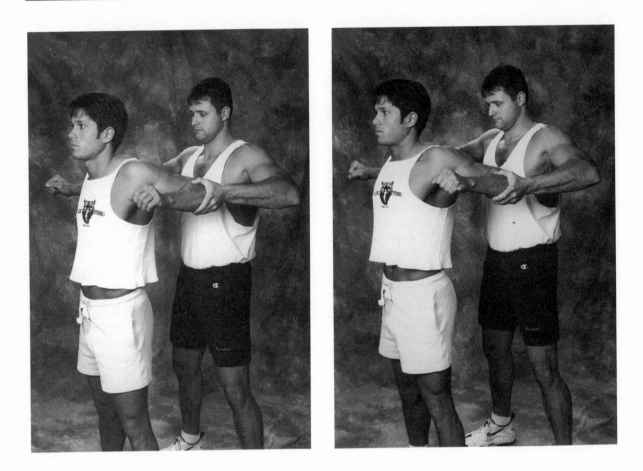

PNF Stretching

Originally conceived as a method of physical therapy, PNF (Pria-neuromuscular facilitation) stretching is performed with a partner who carefully provides resistance for the muscle being stretched prior to actually stretching it. The rationale here is that when you contract a muscle before stretching it, you inhibit the stretch reflex or the body-protective reflex. This reflex prevents you from reaching your potential range of motion. This built-in safety mechanism is set very conservatively. However, "fooling" it through PNF is quite safe when done properly and when you understand your flexibility levels and pain tolerance.

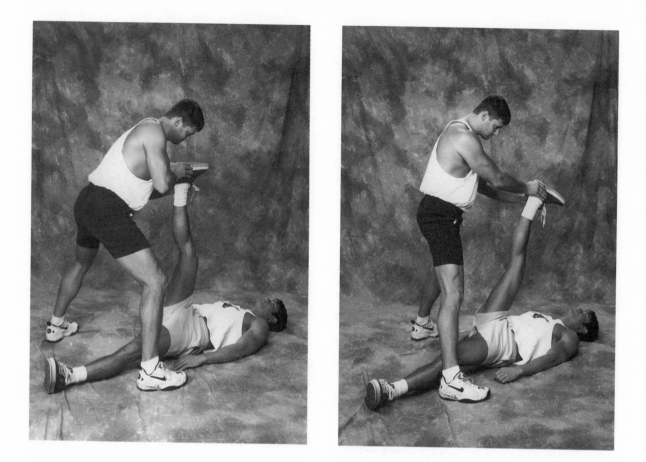

Isometric Stretching

Quite similar to PNF, isometric stretching involves contracting the target muscle against some stationary object prior to stretching it. One example would be spreading your legs into slight discomfort, and then "pinching" your legs into a side-split position to the point of slight discomfort, and then "pinching" your legs toward each other using your abductors (the muscle of your inner thighs). Of course, the resistance offered by the floor will prevent your legs from actually sliding together. After a five-second contraction, relax, and you will find that you will be able to slide further out into the split with no additional discomfort.

At advanced levels, tension can be held for up to thirty seconds. It is advised with this particular exercise that you use something to support yourself should you slip or lose balance. One benefit of this particular stretch is that your adductors become stronger in all ranges of their motion. Keep in mind that the moment you reach a new, higher level of flexibility, you have a small range of that muscle's motion that has never experienced contraction. For this reason, gains in flexibility should be coupled with strength gains in the extreme ranges of motion in order to allay the chances of injury.

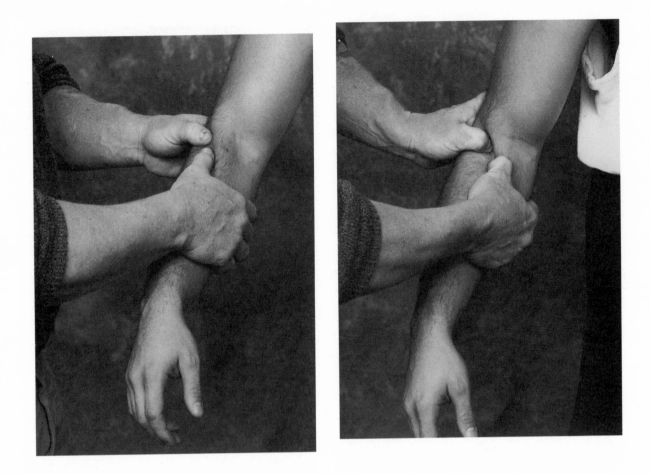

Fascial Stretching

Fascia (the elastic, membranous sheath that encases muscles and muscle groups) can bind and constrict the muscles that surround a joint. Dr. Ida P. Rolf was largely responsible for raising awareness of this phenomenon by developing Structural Ingestion (or Rolfing as it is commonly known), a method of improving the body's natural alignment with gravity by releasing fascial restrictions to allow efficient, natural movements. Fascial stretching involves deep tissue manipulation and should be performed by a competent physical therapist or certified Rolfer. Although fascial stretching is still a new and evolving practice, it holds great promise for those who wish to achieve a permanent increase in their range of motion.

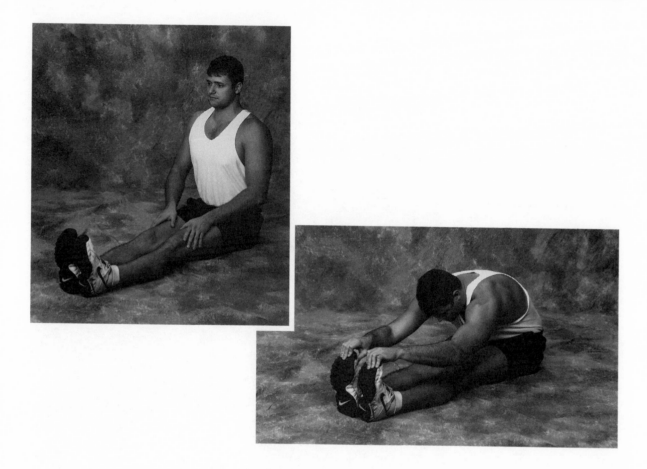

Static Stretching

A slow, gradual, controlled stretch technique through a full range of motion, static stretching is the safest and most universal stretch technique performed. Done correctly, you do the stretching movement until you feel a slight tension, hold that position for about 15 to 25 seconds, breathe out slowly, then try to relax into a slightly deeper stretch. The key word is *relax*. Never bounce or jerk into (or out of) a stretch position.

Be aware that over stretching can cause injury to your body as well. Your body has a safety device that will alert you if you are over stretching. It is called PAIN!

Pain actually tightens the muscle, which is the complete opposite of what you want to accomplish. The catch phrase "No pain, no gain" does *not* apply to stretching. The key is not to have pain, but to relax. The ten basic stretches given in this chapter are examples of static stretching.

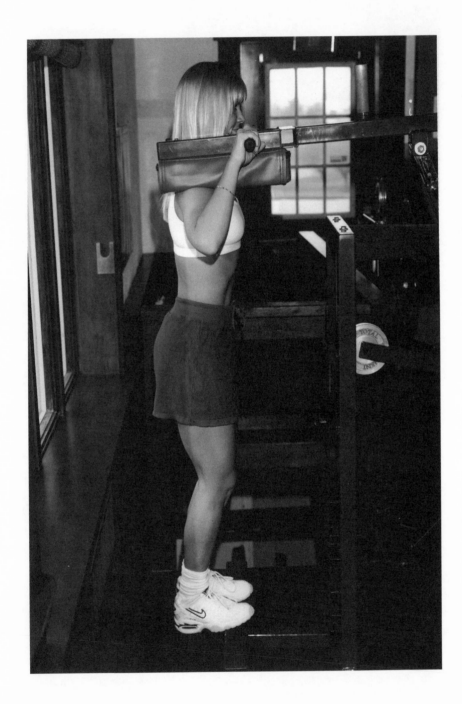

Chapter Five

Beginning Weight Training

By far the most effective way to plan your fitness program is to base it on a combination of aerobic and anaerobic exercise. An examination of just what these two methods of exercise do for the body will explain why I say this.

Aerobic Exercise

Aerobic was a word pretty much confined to the field of cell biology before Kenneth Cooper's groundbreaking books on fitness came out in the 1960s. The message contained in those books, which eventually turned *aerobic* into a universally used synonym for exercise, was simply that you could become as fit as you wanted by systematically intensifying the essential life- and energy-giving process of absorbing oxygen. Based on careful research, Dr. Cooper's instructions for doing this were very straightforward: gradually adapt yourself to sustained movement of large muscle groups at a brisk pace, keep an eye on the rate your heart is beating while you do this, keep it up for at least twenty minutes once you get going, then repeat this at least three times a week.

The stories that started to circulate about how great a person felt after following this prescription soon had people all over the world up and running. They got stitches in their sides of course, but then they had the fun of watching these signs of infirmity disappear as their lungs expanded to do the new work. Non-runners had to listen to runners' reports of ever-increasing times and distances, or less boring, but perhaps more annoying, stories of how running is the perfect exercise, because for a million years our hunter-gatherer ancestors had to chase down their dinner in stone-age grasslands.

Whether or not we actually have a genetic bias toward running—and certainly anyone who has been injured doing it, or just finds it an unpleasant form of exercise, has a right to argue the case—still, Dr. Cooper's prescription for exercise seemed to have made a big impression. How could this be? The statistics on heart disease among middle-aged people at the time were scary, scarier than they are now, and it didn't seem good sense to deliberately stress this "delicate" organ even more. A lot of doctors even had a general policy of advising people over the age of forty to avoid strenuous activity.

People who took this cautious attitude ignored what was so dangerous about a sedentary, physically inactive life. Research was about to prove to them that the oxygen demands of a body at rest, especially a body seated at a demanding desk job, often called for the kind of effort from the heart that could, over time, result in damage to both heart and arteries. The heart is a miraculously strong and durable muscle, contracting at least once for every second of our lives. Under a microscope, its branching, elongated cells and disks are unlike any other tissue in the body. A very intricate network of nerves in its walls ensures that it responds immediately to any signal from the body. Imagine, for instance, somebody in an office job, not very active physically, but still under work pressure.

Because of the low level of physical activity, this person's lungs are moving a minimal amount of air, but the stress of the job is enough to send out signals for more energy-producing oxygen. At this point, the heart steps in with a temporary remedy to save the day: it increases the rate at which it is beating. This is an inefficient but effective way of increasing the amount of oxygen available by increasing the volume of oxygen-saturated blood being pumped. In the end, though, things are not really all that great. The lungs are still operating at way, way below capacity while the heart has been jerked out of slower, stronger beating into a more frequent, weaker pattern of beating—a pattern of strain not untypical of the way our behavior can unproductively turn stress from the outside world into stress for our bodies.

Not that those bodies are totally helpless if asked to handle a little stress. The lungs have an enormous reserve capacity and seem as miraculous as the heart in their ability to stand up to abuse. It's just that the heart and lungs seem complete opposites in the ways they do this. The heart is compact and muscular while the lungs are very different, big, huge in the sheer amount of tissue they contain. Spongy and elastic, they hold large cartilaginous tubes that regress in size to end in the tiniest sacs where, one cell at a time, the red blood cells line up to exchange carbon dioxide for oxygen. Crucially for the lungs of the person we described above, although his lungs sounded like they might be falling down on the job, there is actually nothing at all wrong with them, simply because lungs do not do the job of breathing. This work is done

for them, principally by the perfectly fitted cage of muscle and bone that surrounds them, but ultimately to some degree by all of the voluntary muscles in the body. Our lungs don't move, or don't move much, unless we do.

This is where aerobic exercise comes in: it gets us out of our chairs and moving, so that our heart and lungs together get a chance to stop performing at the low end of their efficiency. By making both organs respond to the demand for oxygen at the same time, aerobic exercise takes the heart and lungs to an entirely different level of functioning. Perhaps the most important benefit from aerobic fitness is that your heart rate at rest, or at a pressured job, will go down by 20,000 to 30,000 beats a day from what it was when you were out of shape. This benefit is only one on a long, well-documented list of reasons for using exercise to flood your body with oxygen. Fat stores are burned up. Resting blood pressure goes down. Energy levels go up. Cholesterol balances improve. The greater volume of blood being pumped both strengthens and increases the number of arteries and capillaries. The kidney, liver, brain, lungs, and skin are cleansed of carbon dioxide and other toxins more thoroughly. The liver increases its production of vital enzymes. Hormone balances are corrected. Four different immune factors are boosted. Aerobic exercise is also widely accepted as a palliative for depression.

Finding a way to fit this type of exercise into your life is made easier by the fact that there are many options to choose from. Walking is popular and is also often recommended by doctors. A gym usually provides a good choice of aerobic machines: stationary bicycles, stair-climbing machines, treadmills, and rowing machines, sometimes even an indoor jogging track. Weight training also provides an excellent way to exercise aerobically. The next chapter, on setting up your program, will explain how aerobic weight training sessions work. Other aerobic exercises include swimming, bicycling, and running.

Target Zone Heart Rate Training

Let's return for a moment to look at one of the instructions in Dr. Cooper's aerobic exercise prescription and spell it out more clearly. I'm talking about his recommendation to keep track of your heart beat during the exercise. The reason for doing this is simple: if you are exercising with the rate too low, you are getting little or no benefit from doing it, and if you are exercising with it too high, you are just causing negative effects. To be more specific, when your heart rate goes out of its target zone on the high end, you are risking heart strain and muscle injury. If your heart is beating at this pace, it will also not be able to meet your body's demand for oxygen. In this state, you can no longer use fat reserves for fuel and have to turn instead to lean muscle mass, pretty much the opposite of what you want to have happen in a workout.

Figure 5-1 will show you the target zone where you want your pulse rate to fall. Your place on the chart is determined by your age and maximum heart rate. The figure the chart uses for maximum heart rate is reached by subtracting your age from 220. The range you want to train in is between 70 percent and 90 percent of this maximum heart rate. If you are forty years old, for instance, a glance at the chart will show you that the target range for your pulse rate is between 126 and 162. When you start exercising, work at the bottom of your range; as you get into better condition, move gradually toward the higher range.

Take your pulse while exercising and immediately afterward. Don't use your thumb and don't press hard. Some people have learned the places where it is easy to get a pulse on their bodies. If you don't know these areas, the wrist and temple are good areas to start. Count the beats for ten seconds (you'll need a watch with a second hand for this) then multiply the figure you get by six. The result is your pulse/heart rate.

Anaerobic Exercise

After hearing about all the benefits conferred by aerobic exercise, up to and including the one where you end up in a permanent good mood, you may have a hard time believing there are things it can't do. But there are, and most of them turn out to be the things that anaerobic exercise can do. As its name signifies, anaerobic exercise is exercise performed without oxygen. Why should anyone want to exercise without oxygen? Some fanatical supporters of aerobic exercise used to ask the question seriously. They also used to point out that the anaerobic effort caused a sudden increase and decrease in blood pressure, not a pattern thought good for the cardiovascular system. It seemed like the kind of thing you would want to avoid if you were trying to be fit. None of these critics suggested outright avoidance, however, perhaps because they knew very well that some very fit athletes—speed skaters, sprint runners, sprint swimmers—train anaerobically. These athletes know that in order to develop the kind of strength they need in their sports, they have to exercise in short, explosive bursts.

The purpose of anaerobic exercise is to develop strength, something it does better than any other form of exercise. Putting an intense, all-out effort into lifting a weight is what you do when you want to stimulate the greatest possible number of muscle fibers. When people began to examine anaerobic exercise more closely, they discovered some previously ignored benefits, like the fact that when muscles are trained for strength this way, they also have much greater endurance than aerobically trained muscles have. Strengthening the skeletal muscles greatly aids the body's balance as well and provides support and stimulation for the circulation of the cardiovascular and lymphatic systems. Anaerobic exercise causes the burning of fat stores in the body for days after you do the exercise. It also strengthens and rejuvenates the major joints of the body, unlike aerobic exercise, which can cause stress and wear to joint cartilage.

Training Heart Rate Target

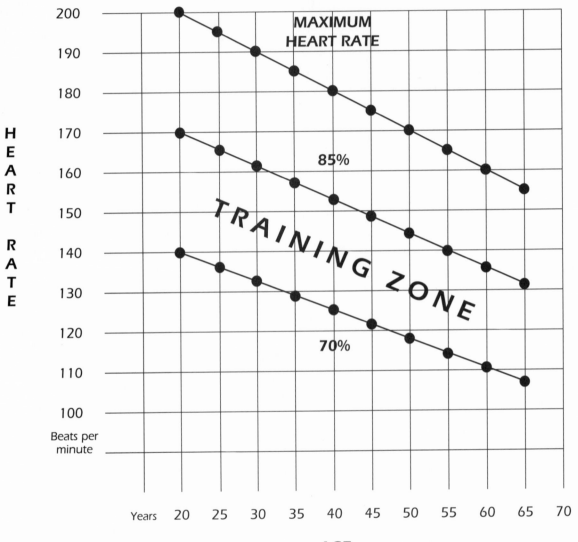

Another important area where anaerobic exercise has more impact than aerobic exercise is the body's rate of metabolism. Your resting metabolic rate goes up and stays up for days after an anaerobic workout. The reason this happens is that the body has to mount a large-scale rebuilding project to repair the tiny tears that develop on muscles during the workout. This same repair project is the reason why anaerobic exercise is so much more effective at causing the development of lean muscle mass than aerobic exercise. Anaerobic exercise is the best stimulant for the replacement of bone mass as well.

It is clear that both of these two forms of exercise are necessary in order to have a truly complete fitness program. Make sure you set up your program with room for both.

The Training Heart Rate Target Chart (above) is adapted from Bruce Algra Fitness Chart Series

Chapter Six

Setting Up Your Program

In your weight training program, you will use special techniques and patterns of movement to lift weight. These techniques are what make it possible to condition and develop your muscles. In normal everyday life, when you pause to lift a weight—let's say it's a dumbbell you want to lift—under direction from your brain your biceps will contract as you raise it, your triceps will contract as you lower it. The contraction of these two muscles starts with nerve impulses acting on tiny muscle fibers, causing them to contract. As you lift the dumbbell just once or twice, nature, in typically efficient manner, uses only a few of the many tiny fibers available in your biceps to get the job done. In weight training, you learn lifting techniques that make it possible to recruit many more of those fibers into the movement of lifting, and test them to their limits while you do it. If you give them time to recover afterward, you will see them gradually turn into larger muscles.

Hypertrophy is the name given to this development of muscle size, and it is known to cause an increase in the muscle's supply of an iron-containing pigment, very similar to hemoglobin, called myoglobin. This substance acts as an oxygen reservoir within the muscle fibers, and an increase in the amount of it available eases the energy-producing work of the muscle cells and greatly increases endurance.

Weight training also has a very direct effect on your entire musculoskeletal system. The stress weight training puts on bones has an effect very much like the effect it has on muscle. It stimulates bone replacement and makes bones stronger, while the same thing is also happening to tendons, ligaments, and cartilage. It even increases the exchange of nutrients between the synovial fluid in bursae, the small sac-like cushions in the joints, and the surrounding cartilage and tendon sheaths.

Reps

The first pattern of movement you learn for weight training is lifting and lowering weights without stopping between lifts until you reach a predetermined number. You are supposed to select the weight you are lifting so you are fairly close to failing by the time you stop. Doing many repetitions of a lift in this measured pattern is called doing reps.

General Fitness

Beginning Weight Training

Maybe weight training is something you think you are not interested in. You may think going to a gym and lifting weights is not for you. Weight training may not be for everybody, but you do not have to be a power lifter or body builder to benefit from basic weight training. You do not even have to touch a barbell! A good weight training program can be designed to suit your fitness needs and requirements, whether it is to tone and trim or to build muscle mass. Modern weight machines offer optimum training for specific muscle groups. Also, working out at a gym gives you the added benefit of expert supervision and advice, plus help and companionship during training efforts. You can get fit on your own . . . but it is easier to do so with friends!

Beginner's Do's and Don't's

1. Before beginning a weight training program, consult your doctor. Inform him of your intentions and get his or her advice about weight training. This is a good rule of thumb before beginning any kind of fitness program, inside or outside a gym.

2. Check our suggestions for proper attire and for the equipment you will need during your weight training program:

   - Cotton warm-up suits
   - Cotton or Lycra shorts
   - T-shirt or muscle shirts
   - Long-sleeve shirts to keep you warm when needed
   - A good pair of cross-training shoes or high-top sneakers
   - A nylon belt rather than a leather belt, for safety and comfort when exercising

3. Choose the time best for you to exercise. Do not exercise immediately after meals. Consuming large amounts of water or eating too close to exercising can limit body fluids and blood supply to the muscles. This can cause dehydration and cramping, because the stomach draws large amounts of these fluids to aid in digestion. Give yourself one to two hours after any meal before weight training.

4. Do not train on an empty stomach. Eat carbohydrates about one to two hours prior to exercising. Remember, carbohydrates are broken down into the fuel the body uses for energy.

5. Drink plenty of water—five to six ounces every fifteen to twenty minutes while you are training.

6. Do not exercise during illnesses.

7. If possible, do not train alone.

8. Set goals for yourself:

   - Use a log book
   - Make your goals short term
   - Keep goals attainable
   - Plan your workouts so you can achieve those goals!

9. Always stretch both before and after your workout.

10. Use weights you can comfortably handle.

11. Perform slow and controlled repetitions using both positive and negative movements. Positive (concentric contraction) movements are those that go from start to finish (lifting) while negative (eccentric contraction) movements go from finish to start (resisting).

Nutrition . . . Stretching . . . Aerobics . . . Weight Training . . .

We have given you some of the basics to get you started on your way to fitness, but that is just the beginning. Now it is time to go into detail. Let's get down to the nitty-gritty of how to set up a program to help you achieve your personal goals with The Winning Factor.

Choosing the Right Weight

This is the variable you need in order to be sure of coming close to failure while still doing the number of reps you want to do. Choose a weight by testing them until you find one that lets you do only two or three extra lifts. If after selecting a weight you cannot do any more reps than your goal, the weight is too heavy. If you can consistently do more than three or four extra reps, the weight is too light.

Sets

You have completed a set when you have done the number of reps you were aiming for and then taken a rest. After the rest, you are ready to repeat the set. The rest period between sets varies from just twenty seconds in aerobic lifting to as long as twenty minutes in anaerobic lifting.

Full Range of Motion

This technique is very important in weight training. It means that in working a muscle, you should take it through its longest possible range of motion. This sounds simple, but when you put it in action you discover there is more to it than this simple description. For one thing, you can't do it as described unless you move slowly, with complete control and awareness. From positive, concentric contraction movements that go from start to finish (lifting) to negative, eccentric contraction movements that go from finish to start (resisting), you will be aware of the involvement of motor neurons with muscle fibers and the alignment and quality of the contraction at every moment.

Breathing

Awareness of the motion of an exercise also includes awareness of your breathing. It's possible to get carried away on this subject. Breathing, of course, is a big part of aerobic exercise, but a conditioned athlete in the middle of a lengthy, repetitive aerobic effort has little temptation to do anything deliberate that runs the risk of interfering with an obviously perfect process that seems to be more than taking care of itself. If you don't happen to be in perfect condition, or if you have a tendency to breathe shallowly, it doesn't hurt to check occasionally to be sure your breath is there. You want to breathe slowly and rhythmically during steady, repetitive exercise.

The single movements done in weight lifting, though, are a different matter. These movements are deliberate enough that you can use your breath to help out in the effort of completing them. This means making a pattern for your breath. Sometimes you take a breath before you begin the exercise. The crunch, or situp, is an example. You take a breath while still prone and motionless, then exhale completely as you begin the movement of sitting up, inhaling again as you lower yourself back to the bench. If you are doing a squat, or knee bend, the pattern can seem different. Here you begin to inhale at the same time you bend your knees to begin the exercise, then you exhale at the end of the bend as you begin to return to an upright or straight position. Though you begin to inhale at different points in these two exercises, the basic pattern still remains the same, as it remains the same for pretty much all of the exercises. The simple guideline to follow is to breathe in during the more relaxed part of the exercise and breathe out with effort. Take complete breaths, starting deep in the diaphragm and using both nose and mouth to take in air. Always remember to exhale, and do it completely, explosively if that helps.

When stressed, some people have a tendency to stop, or almost stop, breathing. There is a very serious rule against holding your breath in weight training. The squat/knee bend mentioned above is a good exercise to illustrate the reason for this rule. When you start the effort of rising from a squat, you will naturally contract your diaphragm muscle to help the other muscles you are using.

TABLE 6-1

Levels of Conditioning in Aerobic Weight Training		
LOW-REP AEROBIC WEIGHT TRAINING		
Week	Number of Reps per Exercise	Number of Sets per Exercise
1	20	3
2	25	3
3	30	3
MEDIUM-REP AEROBIC WEIGHT TRAINING		
1	35	2
2	40	2
3	45	2
HIGH-REP AEROBIC WEIGHT TRAINING		
1	50	1
2	55	1
3	60	1

When the diaphragm contracts, it presses up into the chamber holding your lungs, just as it does when you breathe out. If you actually can manage to hold your breath at this point, you run a real risk of injury, probably to tissue in the area of the epiglottis, the flap of cartilage that closes your throat to air when you swallow or hold your breath. So you have two reasons for breathing in deliberate patterns during weight training: primarily it assists you in getting your complete energy into the movements of the exercises, but at the same time it keeps you from accidentally holding your breath.

Aerobic Weight Training

Aerobic weight training requires a high number of reps, performed with short rests between sets. To a degree, it develops cardiovascular endurance like other aerobic exercises, but because you can also progressively increase the weights you use in the exercises, you will be able to develop more lean mass on average than you will with the other forms of aerobic exercise. Table 6-1 outlines an aerobic program with three levels of conditioning.

Anaerobic Weight Training

Anaerobic weight training uses a short, intense burst of energy in lifting. Its purpose is to build absolute strength, the kind of strength that makes everything else you do seem easy. When doing a lower number of reps, starting with just one, movements can be explosive—that is, starting slowly, then accelerating. Rests between sets are long. At higher reps, going up to fifteen, movements can be moderate and rest periods correspondingly shorter. Table 6-2 below gives you an idea of the range of anaerobic workouts and shows how the weight is to be adjusted between low-rep and high-rep sessions. The percentages are to be taken of the maximum weight you can lift once.

TABLE 6-2

Anaerobic Weight Training

CHOICE 1: VERY HEAVY WEIGHT		
Sets per exercise	Reps per Set	Percentage of Maximum Weight
6	1–2	95
6	3	90
6	4	85
CHOICE 2: HEAVY WEIGHT		
5	5	80
5	6	75
5	8	70
CHOICE 3: MODERATE HEAVY WEIGHT		
4	10	65
4	12	60
4	15	55

Goals

Make your goals short and attainable, and write them down. A log book is an indispensable aid for keeping track of your progress as you work toward your goals. Buy one that will hold plenty of information, including photos. Start by writing down your entire program, then go on to keep a complete diary of your training sessions and diet. Memory can play tricks on you if you don't keep a record.

Avoid Injuries

- Always stretch both before and after your workout.
- Use weights you can comfortably handle.
- Don't exercise when you are ill.
- Don't exercise alone if you don't have to.

Keep Your Stomach Happy While You Work Out

Choose the time you like best to exercise, but be careful not to make it immediately after a meal. The digestive process is complex and makes a big demand on the body's blood and lymph supply. If you try to work out when your stomach is full and hard at work, you start a conflict in your cardiovascular system, calling for excess blood and fluid in too many places at once. Dehydration can result along with a variety of unpleasant conditions, from nausea to cramps.

On the other hand, don't try to train on too empty a stomach. Being too depleted of food means your glycogen reserves won't hold up to give you the energy you need. Take some carbohydrates about one to two hours before exercising to keep this from happening.

Drink plenty of water, five to six ounces every fifteen to twenty minutes while you are training.

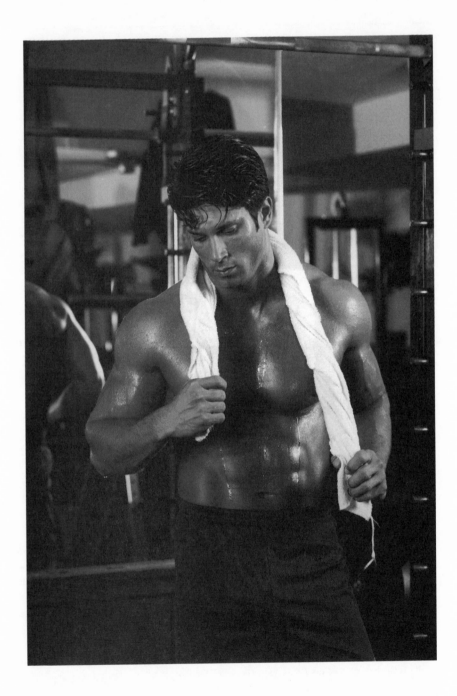

Chapter Seven

Overtraining

If you are doing weight training, your fitness program has built-in intensity. As you move through repetitions and sets, adjustments are made to the weight resistance you are handling in order to keep pace with your body's growing strength. The special programs for weight loss or weight gain depend on intensity for success. And, of course, everyone adds their own degree of intensity to the exercises, especially in the beginning, when they discover how much fun it can be to do them. Some of these people like to go on increasing the pace for adding resistance or adding workout time by reducing rest time.

Be prepared, though: you may wake up one day and find that the enjoyment that was making you so gung ho seems to have gone out the window. A dull what-am-I-doing-here feeling has replaced the excitement you used to have about getting at the weights in the gym. Perhaps you even look haggard and thin, and those hours of deep, refreshing sleep that seemed to be an almost automatic reward for doing a good, heavy workout have been replaced by hours of insomnia.

Any of the above problems can be a sign that you have been overtraining. The list of warning signals can also include a depressed immune system that suddenly becomes prone to colds or flu, lack of appetite, or constant soreness. You don't even have to be that gung ho to cause some or all of these things. Take the soreness, for instance.

There are two kinds: one is a symptom of overtraining, but some soreness is also a natural result of the anaerobic part of your routine. Lifting weights anaerobically causes some microtrauma to the muscles. One product of the breakdown phase of this trauma is an amino acid carrying hydrogen ions, hydroxyproline. It takes about twenty-four to forty-eight hours to disperse in the body, but it is caustic enough to cause plenty of irritation to nerve endings in muscle when it does reach them. Called delayed onset muscle soreness (DOMS), its effects can often be controlled by adjusting your program, possibly by increasing the intensity of the cardio-respiratory exercises in your sessions to make them more efficient in removing toxins and wastes from your body.

Probably the first thing you should do when you experience symptoms of overtraining—particularly if they are not that severe, or mostly consist of sudden onset fatigue—is take a close look at how you are eating. Honestly examine how faithfully you have been following the nutrition guidelines. Check if you are eating enough, and especially if you are balancing carbohydrates and proteins, spacing them out in five or six small meals during the day. Because of the demands exercise makes on your body, fatigue-causing insulin imbalances can arise very quickly if you start neglecting your nutrition.

If after checking your diet you decide overtraining is the cause of your problems, start working on a solution by remembering that rest has to be an integral part of your weight training program. The more intensely you train, the more recuperation time your body needs to rest and rebuild itself. The sessions described in this book are always to be spaced out between two and five times a week. Keep your training in a rhythm, consistently alternating workout days with rest days, as I recommend for a particular program. If you don't do this, you will simply be defeating your efforts to be fit because you will actually be breaking down lean body mass rather than increasing it. Following is a list of further suggestions for dealing with overtraining. Most of these suggestions will also have some effect in lessening DOMS as well.

1. Look for ways to reduce the level of intensity in the workouts. For instance, simply reduce the number of sets and reps. Or, if you do not want to reduce the length of time you spend in your sessions, you can split the assignment of the exercises so that one day you work just the chest and back, say, and work the shoulders and arms another day, the thighs and calves a third. If you have been regularly picking days when you go all out for maximum effort in a session, make certain that you have at least a week's space between these days. One trick you can use to reduce the risk of overtraining is to avoid doing negatives. Negatives are exercises done using weights that are too heavy; you can perform the negative part of the exercise, but not the positive part (without the assistance of spotters). Negatives are popular among some advanced athletes, but more times than not the technique results in overtraining, because of the tremendous amount of cellular damage negatives create.

2. Make sure you are using good lifting technique. This means slowly and smoothly completing movements through a full range of motion, without contorting your body. You will typically tend to sacrifice good lifting form if you try to use too much weight. Doing this forces you to try to bring in extraneous muscles to help out the ones more directly involved in the exercise, a process appropriately called cheating. Another form of cheating, also to be avoided, is called ballistic lifting, the word *ballistic* indicating that the weight's resistance more than the lifter's control is determining the trajectory of the lift. Good technique requires controlled lifting.

3. Besides checking your diet in general, as I suggested above, also check your vitamin/mineral supplementation, and investigate the list of supplements in chapter 3 for one that might work best for you.

4. Practice a healthy lifestyle by avoiding alcohol, tobacco, and recreational drugs.

5. Allow time for plenty of rest between workouts, and consider making time for one or two twenty-minute catnaps during the day.

6. Take advantage of various therapeutic modalities, such as whirlpools, saunas, heat, ice, massage, etc.

7. Take advantage of the extra power your mind can provide for your workouts. Make it a regular part of your routine to visualize yourself performing an exercise before you perform it. Mentally rehearsing a movement this way can give you a surprisingly strong boost of energy. Many people also find that setting aside some time every day for meditation lowers stress and makes it easier to stay focused.

8. Always remember good common sense. If you feel you are fatigued and sore enough to justify it, don't hesitate to cut back on your program, or stop it entirely for a while, to give yourself some plain old rest. Sensing when to do this can be an important part of eventually reaching your goals.

Chapter Eight

Weight Training for Fat Loss

One of the most popular and attainable goals in weight training is to give your body an overall thinner, leaner look. This chapter has an exercise program that will help you achieve this goal, but before we get to it I want to talk again about the important part nutrition plays in this program and in all the programs in this book. Perhaps like many of the people who come to my gym, you are trying to follow one of the conventional weight-reduction diets, or have tried to follow such a diet in the past. If you have, I want you to know that there are several important differences between this program for fat loss and the standard weight loss diets most people try to follow.

The first difference is in the use of the word *fat* instead of *weight* to describe the loss. When you do this program, you end up with a thinner, leaner look because you have reduced unwanted reserves of fat. On conventional diets, if you get a leaner look, it is the result of what can technically be called emaciation. Emaciation is an accurate description of the wasting-away process these diets trigger, especially the diets that bring quick results you can measure by getting on your scale. All of these diets call for a drastic reduction of one or more of the three essential food groups: protein, carbohydrates, or fats. Starving the body this way, at a minimum, robs it of energy, while in the case of low-carbohydrate diets, usually the most popular, it dehydrates the body extensively, resulting in the

removal of essential nutrients and a drastic reduction of water in the muscle cells. Perhaps a more important disadvantage of these diets for someone who is trying to be fit is the way they trigger the body's catabolic function so that as much as 50 percent of the weight you lose by following them comes from the direct loss of muscle mass.

When you diet conscientiously enough to bring about a quick loss of weight, you are merely setting off a signal to your body's very effective system for maintaining internal equilibrium. In this case, one of the things this system does is send a signal for a special fat storage enzyme to go to work stockpiling as much fat as possible. Once triggered, this fat enzyme stays at work for some time, almost always long enough to be still hard at work wanting to store fat when you finally give in to your hunger and decide you can start eating again. This is the familiar yo-yo effect of dieting, and as well as being completely counterproductive, it can also be seriously unhealthy.

A person who chooses to lose fat in a weight training program has to avoid the unhealthy pitfalls of dieting. The reason for this is simple: you have to have adequate nutrition to keep up with the exercises. When you do weight training, you are continually working at increasing the amount of energy you use. Since your metabolism provides this energy from food, you need to continually feed more calories to your metabolism. The fact is you have to eat when you are in a weight training program or you won't reach any of your goals, and that includes fat loss.

The training for the fat loss program allows for some reduction of calorie intake, if you are certain this can be done with balance and moderation, without any intention of getting instant results. The worst mistake you can make is to try to lose fat in a hurry and end up cutting too many calories. Think of the whole process as happening over years rather than months, and never in weeks. Just work to make your developing muscles into super fat-burners while they grow to increase your body's percentage of lean mass. At the same time, the many small meals you are taking will also gradually lower your homeostatic set point so that you will be confident that whatever fat you lose will stay lost. Losing inches in the places you want to lose them is what counts.

The guidelines you have to follow for your nutrition are based on the three essential food groups. Protein comes first. Your body needs protein for repair and maintenance of muscle tissue, in particular the tissue you break down in regular exercise. The amino acids that result when protein is broken down can also be used for producing energy. When you are not getting enough protein, your metabolism will start breaking down the valuable existing muscle you have just worked so hard to maintain, or increase, to use it for protein. It is therefore very important to calculate your requirement for protein so there is enough to fully support your program goals.

Once you establish your protein needs, you can figure your quotas for carbohydrate and fat. Both of these nutrients supply energy directly—fat for the long haul—while carbohydrates are especially important to answer immediate demands. You also need to eat enough carbohydrates to aid in absorbing and metabolizing protein. (See table 2–3 on page 9 for information on balancing fats, carbohydrates, and protein.)

Fat is consumed for energy during exercise only when a lot of oxygen is present. Aerobic exercise, then, is the obvious choice to lead a fat-loss program. The continuous performance of high-rep aerobic lifting, with short, less-than-a-minute rests between sets, gets a high blood transport of fat-burning oxygen going. It also brings on a sharp increase in the body's production of fat-burning enzymes and in the end develops longer, leaner muscles. As you become more fit, you can take advantage of aerobic exercise's positive cycle of increasing capacity to raise the intensity of these workouts. The result will be a corresponding increase in the percentage of fat reserves that are lost.

Aerobic weight training gets priority in shaping your program for fat loss, but this does not mean you should ignore anaerobic workouts. They provide a perfect complement to aerobic lifting by causing fat stores to burn when you are not exercising. The increase in muscle tissue that anaerobic lifting causes in turn brings on both a greatly increased rate of metabolism and the release of the powerful fat-burning growth hormone. Getting in some anaerobic workouts will help a lot in keeping your percentage of lean mass high and will guarantee that you are burning fat around the clock. Remember, though, that if you are able to raise the intensity of your aerobic sessions and add some anaerobic lifting, you have two more reasons to keep a close watch on your nutrition. You are developing calorie-burning, metabolically active muscle. You have to provide enough food or your muscle tissue will be sacrificed in its place in the metabolic process.

TABLE 8-1

Endurance Progressive Program for Fat Loss and Lean Mass Maintenance

Day	Exercise	Sets
1	Squat Or Leg Press	3
	Hack Squat	2
	Leg Curl	2
	Leg Extension	2
	Lunge with Weight	2
	Calf	2
	Leg Raise	2
	Crunch	2
2	Chest and Bench Press	3
	Shoulder or Military Press	2
	Seated Long Row	2
	Low Back or Stiff Deadlift	2
	Bicep Curl	2
	Tricep Press or Extension	2
	Leg Raise	2
	Crunch	2

Week	Number of Reps
1 and 2	10 very slow 15 explosive
3 and 4	30 medium reps
5 and 6	15 very slow 20 explosive
7 and 8	40 medium reps

This sample program works well for fat loss, taking nutritional aspects into consideration. It is a highly intense eight-week weight training program, with three days each week spent doing cardiovascular work and two days using weight machines (see chapter 13 for instructions on the exercises). I suggest taking weekends off. Work on weight training Tuesdays and Thursdays and spend Mondays, Wednesdays, and Fridays doing cardiovascular exercise for forty to sixty minutes. Make sure you keep your heart rate in the target zone. See Heart Rate Target Chart on page 48.

*Pictured is Dr. Job Menges, M.D.
As an orthopedic surgeon, he is
one of many physicians beginning
to understand the importance of
nutrition, supplementation, and
exercise. Dr. Menges came to John
for exercise, nutrition, and
supplementation advice prior to
his hip replacement surgery. Only
three weeks after the operation,
Job was back in the gym using
John's training and nutritional
recommendations to maintain an
outstanding 11 percent body fat
level at sixty-three years of age.*

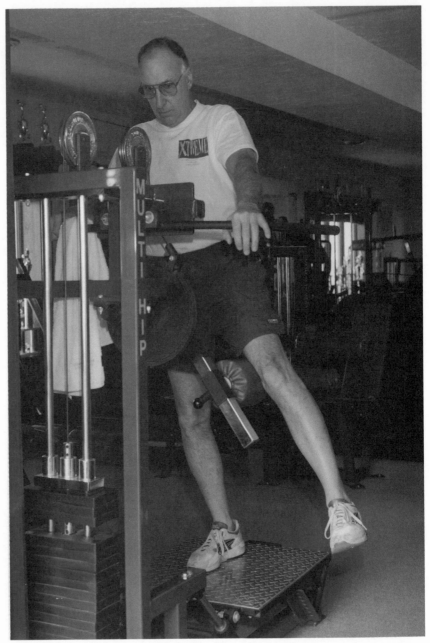

Chapter Nine

Weight Training for Weight Gain

In weight gain, just as in weight loss, your goal involves much more than just numbers on a scale. Your goal in weight gain should be to increase your lean mass without any gain in body fat. The key to this, once again, is proper nutrition. You must increase your calorie consumption, but it is when you eat and what you eat rather than simply how much you eat that makes the difference. You will be using the zig-zag method we discussed in chapter 2. This means eating carbohydrate-rich meals to store energy before the workouts, and protein-rich meals for recovery after workouts.

Your protein intake should be as high as 0.9 to 1.0 grams per pound of lean muscle mass, but do not exceed thirty grams per serving, because in most cases your body simply cannot absorb more than that every three hours. Your carbohydrates must increase also. The calories should balance out at approximately forty percent protein, forty-five percent carbohydrates, and fifteen percent fat. Remember that the amount of protein you consume should be based on your body's needs as determined by your lean mass.

Your workout regime will also dictate your carbohydrate and fat consumption. Lean mass weight gains come from exercise and recovery repeated over and over again. Use pin-point timing as far as rests between workouts and the best time for meals. Total body weight may be increased by the random consumption of large amounts of calories, but pure muscle gains are another matter. You may be very surprised at the size of the lean mass gains that can be made through timing of minimum calories rather than the ransom consumption of mega-calories. Timing of intake is far more important than total calorie consumption when it comes to lean mass gains.

Here are two recommended ways to gain lean mass through weight training:

- Anaerobic power, where you use overloading in the workouts, working with predominantly white, fast-twitch muscle fiber and progressive increase in weight.
- Both anaerobic and aerobic power, where you use both white, fast-twitch muscle and red, slow-twitch muscle. This method is the fastest way to gain lean mass.

Your muscle is composed of two types of muscle fibers: red, slow-twitch fibers are used for endur-

TABLE 9-1

Sample Four-Day Bodybuilding Program for Weight Gain Through Lean Mass

Day	Exercise	Sets
1	Bench Press	4
	Camber Bench Press	3
	Reverse Bench Press	3
	Shoulder Press	3
	French Curl	3
	Tricep Machine	3
	Tricep Pushdown	3
2	Squat	4
	Leg Press	4
	Hack Squat	3
	Leg Extension	3
	Leg Curl	3
	Standing Curl	4
	Seated Calf	3
	Plus any three of the following:	
	Bar Curls of Choice	4
	Bicep Machine	4
	Dumbbell Curl	4
	Concentration Curl	3
3	Incline Bench Press	4
	Decline Bench Press	4
	Military Press Lateral Raise	4
	Rear Raise	3
	Any two Triceps Exercises	2
4	Stiff Leg Deadlift	3
	Bent Row	4
	One-arm Dumbbell Row	3
	Vertical or Seat Row	3
	Camber Bar Trap Shrug	4
	Front Lateral Pull	4
	Any two Bicep Exercises	2

TABLE 9-1 (CONTINUED)

Sample Four-Day Bodybuilding Program for Weight Gain Through Lean Mass

Week	Number of Reps
1–3	15
4–6	12
7–9	10
10–12	8

Work with your abdominals two to three days a week, up to a total of twelve per day. You should use 65 percent of your maximum weight for all the above sets, and always be sure to warm up.

Hints for Weight Gain

- Controlling fat intake is still important on a weight program, although not as critical as it is on a weight-reduction program.
- A weight gain program is usually accompanied by a more strenuous workout; greater fat intake is necessary for energy.
- Low-cholesterol margarine, peanut butter, and cheeses can be added to the above menus when fat intake needs to be increased to meet guidelines.
- Select five meals per day from the menus in chapter 2, doubling the breakfast, lunch, and dinner portions. Add pre- and post-workout meal with unlimited snacks.
- Powdered supplements can be added to beverages to increase the nutritional value of your snacks.
- Pre-workout meals should be high in complex carbohydrates.
- Post-workout meals should be high in proteins (25–30 grams).
- Your total caloric intake for weight gain will vary according to your individual lean mass and should probably not exceed 5,000 calories with no more than 45 grams of fat.

Hints for Fat Loss

- Increase your body heat by combining your exercise with frequent meals—five to six small meals a day. The resulting heat-generating effect on the body is called *thermogenesis*.
- Do resistance exercise to increase lean mass—the more lean mass, the more calories you burn.
- Avoid dieting that involves not eating, starving, or fasting. This causes your fat cells to become more efficient at storing fat and causes your calorie-burning ability to become less efficient.
- Eat to lose body fat. Contrary to what people think, if you do not take in enough calories, your metabolism slows down, which in turn makes it much harder to lose fat.

ance and burn fat for energy, and white, fast-twitch fibers are called into play for strength and power and use both glycogen and fat for energy.

Table 9-1 is a sample four-day bodybuilding mass program that uses mostly white fiber. The table doesn't show the warm-ups, but they should be adapted to your needs; don't skip them. In your warm-ups, use lighter weights, increasing through three to five sets until you reach your goal weight. After your warm-up, do all of your sets at your goal weight, which should be 65 to 85 percent of your maximum.

Now here is a twist for you. Table 9-2 provides a three-week program, training just two days a week, with reps increasing each week. At first glance, this looks like a high-rep aerobic program, but in reality it is still an anaerobic weight training program. We have achieved incredible lean mass gains in just a three-week period with this program, using red, intermediate, and white muscle fiber. We might use this program every eight to twelve weeks, or after a low-rep, heavier-weight training cycle. It provides a great base on which to start or end your cycle training. Give it a try—you might be surprised at the results.

Remember, always finish with explosive movements, movements that begin slowly and then accelerate through the lift. This is a very good technique for activating motor neurons in white fiber, high-strength muscle. Reps are split in each set. The first half of the reps should be performed very slowly on both positive and negative movements; take approximately 3.5 seconds on both concentric and eccentric (positive and negative) movements. The second half of the reps should be controlled as you do eccentric, or negative, movements, and explosive on the concentric, or positive, movements. Always use moderate control on negative movements and maximum acceleration on positive. In attempting explosive movements, do not allow them to become ballistic. Ballistic movements are what happens when the weight begins to control you. For instance, when you have to bounce it to lift it, or if in lifting it you send it on a trajectory where you are not confident about the outcome.

A word of caution: Because of the amount of microtrauma to the muscles that this program produces in a short time, do not use it for more than three weeks.

TABLE 9-2

Two-Day Program for Endurance and Increasing Lean Mass

Day	Exercise	Sets
1	Squats and/or Leg Press	3
	Hack Squat	2
	Leg Curl	2
	Leg Extension	2
	Lunge with Weight	2
	Calf	2
	Leg Raise	2
	Crunch	2
2	Chest or Bench Press	3
	Shoulder or Military Press	2
	Seated Long Row	2
	Low Back or Stiff Leg Deadlift	2
	Bicep Curl	2
	Tricep Press or Extension	2
	Leg Raise	2
	Crunch	2

Week	Number of Reps
1	10 Very Slow (3.5 Sec)
	10 Explosive
2	10 Very Slow (3.5 Sec)
	10 Explosive
3	15 Very Slow (3.5 Sec)
	15 Explosive

Very slow reps should take about 3.5 seconds. For a good way to judge what amount of weight to use, if you can do 2 or 3 extra reps, your weight is about right. If you cannot do any more reps than your goal, you are too heavy. If you can do more than 4 or 5 extra reps, you are too light.

Chapter Ten

Exercise Programs for Sports

TABLE 10-1

Beginning General Conditioning		
Days	Exercises	Number of Reps
1 and 3	Warm-Up Bike	10
	Leg Curls	10
	Leg Press	10
	Leg Raise	10
	Crunch	10
2 and 4	Vertical Row	10
	Lat Machine	10
	Shoulder Press	10
	Pec Deck	10
	Chest Press	10
	Bicep Machine	10
	Tricep Machine	10
	Lower Back	10
	Leg Raise	10
	Crunch	10

Weeks	Number of Sets
1 and 2	1
3 and 4	2
5 and 6	3
7 and 8	4

Beginning General Conditioning

This is an excellent program for beginners to follow. Before you begin training, here are some things to keep in mind.

1. Always see a doctor, have a physical examination, and let him know your intentions and the type of exercise you plan on doing.
2. Start a new exercise program with moderation and build up through the program slowly.
3. Use weights you can comfortably handle while performing slow and controlled repetitions.
4. Always stretch before and after your workout.

TABLE 10-2

Four-Day Bodybuilding Mass

Day	Exercise	Number of Sets	Number of Sets
1	Bench Press	4	15
	Camber Bench Press	3	8
	Reverse Bench Press	3	8
	Shoulder Press	2	8
Plus any three of the following:			
	French Curl	4	12
	Dips with Weight	4	8
	Tricep Machine	4	8
	Tricep Push Down	4	8
2	Squats	4	15
	Leg Press	3	8
	Hack Squat	3	8
	Leg Extension	2	8
	Leg Curl	3	8
	Standing Calf	4	15
	Seated Calf	2	15
	Bicep Machine	4	8
	Dumbbell	4	8
	Concentration Curl	2	15
3	Incline Bench Press	4	8
	Decline Bench Press	4	8
	Military Press	4	8
	Lateral Raise	3	8
	Rear Raise	3	8
	Any two Tricep Exercises	2	8
4	Stiff Leg Deadlift	3	15
	Bent Row	4	8
	One-arm Dumbbell Row	3	8
	Vertical or Seat Row	3	8
	Camber Bar Trap Shrug	3	8
	Front Lat Pull	4	8
	Any two Bicep Exercises	2	15

Bodybuilding Mass

1. Abdominals are worked two to three days a week up to twelve sets total per day.
2. This program does not include warm-up sets. Make sure you warm up first.
3. Use the same weights for all sets. They should be 75 to 85 percent of your maximum.

TABLE 10-3

Tennis		
Day	Exercise	Number of Sets
1 and 3	Squat or Leg Press	4
	Hack Squat	4
	Leg Extension	4
	Leg Curl	4
	Standing Calf	4
	Lunge with Weight	4
2	Chest Press or Bench Press	4
	Shoulder or Military Press	4
	Front Deltoid Raise	4
	Side Lateral Raise	4
	Dumbbell Swing *	3
	Dumbbell Swing **	3
	Dumbbell Swing ***	3
	Bicep Curl Machine	2
	Tricep Machine	2
	Leg Raise	3
	Crunch	2

Week	Number of Reps
1 and 2	15
3 and 4	20
5 and 6	25
7 and 8	30

   * Forehand stroke, both arms
  ** Backhand stroke, both arms
*** Serve both arms

Tennis Instructions

1. Always see a doctor, have a physical examination, and let him know your intentions and the type of exercise you plan on doing.
2. Start a new exercise program with moderation and build up through the program slowly.
3. This program is designed as an eight-week program, but can be extended for up to ten or twelve weeks by adding one week per weekly interval beginning with weeks one and two.
4. Use weights you can comfortably handle while performing slow and controlled positive movements. The negative movements should be twice as slow.
5. Always stretch before and after your workout.
6. This program should be done two to three days per week with a minimum of one day of rest between each workout.
7. When performing lunges with weight, never put weight on your shoulders because of the risk of injury to the lower back. Hold the dumbbells in your hands and let them hang at your sides.
8. Dumbbell swings are performed slowly in a controlled manner to improve your strength through a full range of motion. Never swing with fast or jerky movements.

TABLE 10-4

Golf

Day	Exercise	Number of Sets
1 and 3	Chest Press or Bench Press	4
	Shoulder or Military Press	3
	Vertical or Long Row	3
	Front Lat Pull	3
	Toe Touches with Dumbbell*	4
	Golf Swing with Dumbbell on right side	4
	Golf Swing with Dumbbell on Left Side	4
	Bicep Machine	3
	Tricep Machine	3
2	Squat or Leg Press	4
	Hack Squat	3
	Leg Extension	3
	Leg Curl	3
	Standing Calf	3
	Leg Raise	3
	Crunch	3

Week	Number of Reps
1 and 2	16
3 and 4	18
5 and 6	20
7 and 8	22

* Left hand to right foot and right hand to left foot

Golf Instructions

Golf swings are performed in a slow and controlled manner through a full range of motion to improve strength. Swings should never be fast or jerky.

1. Always see a doctor, have a physical examination, and let him know your intentions and the type of exercise you plan on doing.
2. Start a new exercise program with moderation and build up through the program slowly.
3. This program is designed as an eight-week program, but can be extended for up to ten or twelve weeks by adding one week per weekly interval beginning with weeks one and two.
4. Use weights you can comfortably handle while performing slow and controlled positive movements. The negative movements should take twice as long as the positive ones.
5. Always stretch before and after your workout.
6. This program may be utilized two to three days per week with a minimum of one day of rest between each workout.

TABLE 10-5

Football (off season)

Day	Exercise	Number of Sets
1	Front Squat	4
	Leg Press	4
	Hack Squat	3
	Leg Curl	2
	Leg Extension	2
	Standing Calf	3
2	Chest or Bench Press (Wide Grip)	3
	Chest or Bench Press (Close Grip)	3
	Shoulder Press Front	2
	Shoulder Press Rear	2
	Tricep Push Down	3
	Bicep Curl	3
	Hanging Leg Raise	4
	Leg Tuck	4
	Crunches	3
3	Hang Clean	4
	Stiff Leg Deadlift	2
	Long Row	2
	Vertical Row	2
	Shrug	2
	Bent Row	2
	Front Lat Pull	2
	Hanging Leg Raise	4
	Leg Tuck (Bench)	4
	Crunches	3

Week	Number of Reps
1 and 2	8
3 and 4	10
5 and 6	12
7 and 8	15

Football Instructions

1. Always see a doctor, have a physical examination, and let him know your intentions and the type of exercise you plan on doing.
2. Start a new exercise program with moderation and build up through the program slowly.
3. This program is designed as an eight-week program, but can be extended for up to ten or twelve weeks by adding one week per weekly interval beginning with weeks one and two.
4. Use weights you can comfortably handle while performing slow and controlled positive movements. The negative movements should be twice as slow.
5. Always stretch before and after your workout.
6. This program is three days per week with a minimum of one day of rest between each workout.
7. All running and sprinting should be done on off days of weight training.

TABLE 10-6

Baseball

Day	Exercise	Number of Sets (x Extra Reps)
1	Chest Press	4
	Chest Press Downset	1 x 14
	Shoulder Press	4
	Pec Deck	4
	Tricep Machine	4
	Tricep Push Down	4
	Baseball Swing Dumbbell, Both Arms	4
	Twist	2 x 20
	Good Morning	2 x 20
2	Leg Press	4
	Leg Extension	4
	Leg Curl	4
	Leg Raise	2 x 20
	Crunch	2 x 20
3	Stiff Leg Deadlift	4
	Stiff Leg Deadlift Downset	1 x 14
	Bent Row	4
	Seat Row	4
	Shrug	4
	Front Lat Pull	4
	Baseball Swing	4
	Baseball Throw	4

Week	Number of Reps
1 and 2	6
3 and 4	8
5 and 6	10
7 and 8	15

Baseball Instructions

1. Always see a doctor, have a physical examination, and let him know your intentions and the type of exercise you plan on doing.
2. Start a new exercise program with moderation and build up through the program slowly.
3. This program is designed as an eight-week program, but can be extended for up to ten or twelve weeks by adding one week per weekly interval beginning with weeks one and two.
4. Use weights you can comfortably handle while performing slow and controlled positive movements. The negative movements should take twice as long as the positive ones.
5. Always stretch before and after your workout.
6. This program should be done two to three days per week with a minimum of one day of rest between each workout.
7. Downsets are exercises that use 25 percent less weight than used on the main exercise.
8. Baseball swings and throws are performed slowly and are controlled through a full range of motion to improve strength; they should never be fast or jerky.

TABLE 10-7

Basketball (off season)		
Day	**Exercise**	**Number of Sets**
1	Leg Press	4
	Leg Press Downset	1 x 25
	Hack Squat	4
	Leg Extension	4
	Leg Curl	4
	Standing Calf	4
	Seated Calf	4
	Baseball Throw	4
	Bench Leg Raise	4 x 10
	Chair Leg Raise	4 x 10
	Crunches	4 x 10
2	Chest Press	4
	Chest Press Downset	1 x 25
	Shoulder Press Front	4
	Shoulder Press Rear	4
	Bicep Machine	4
	Tricep Machine	4
	Tricep Press-Down	4
	Dips	4
	Dumbbell Twist	4
3	Stiff Leg Deadlift*	4
	Stiff leg Deadlift Downset	1 x 25
	Bent Row	4
	Seat Row	4
	Leg Extension	4
	Vertical Row	4
	Shrug	4
	Front Lat Pull	4
	Bench Leg Raise	4 x 10
	Chair Leg Raise	4 x 10
	Crunches	4 x 10

Week	Number of Reps
1 and 2	8
3 and 4	10
5 and 6	12
7 and 8	15

*Start 3 inches below the knee with knees slightly bent

Basketball Instructions

1. Always see a doctor, have a physical examination, and let him know your intentions and the type of exercise you plan on doing.
2. Start a new exercise program with moderation and build up through the program slowly.
3. This program is designed as an eight-week program, but can be extended for up to ten or twelve weeks by adding one week per weekly interval beginning with weeks one and two.
4. Use weights you can comfortably handle while performing slow and controlled positive movements. The negative movements should be twice as slow.
5. Always stretch before and after your workout.
6. This program is three days per week with a minimum of one day of rest between each workout.
7. Downsets are always 25 percent less weight than used on the main exercise.
8. Dumbbell twists are performed in a slow and controlled manner. Your right arm is extended fully to the right side and the left arm is bent so the left hand is over the right pectoral. The left side is performed the opposite way of the right side.

TABLE 10-8

Soccer		
Day	Exercise	Number of Sets (x Extra Reps)
1	Leg Press	4
	Leg Press Downset	1 x 25
	Hack Squat	4
	Leg Extension	4
	Shrug	4
	Leg Curl	4
	Standing Calf	4
	Leg Raise	4 x 12
	Crunch	4 x 12
	Good Morning	4 x 12
2	Chest Press	4
	Chest Press Downset	1 x 25
	Shoulder Press, Front	4
	Shoulder Press, Rear	4
	Shrug	4
	Tricep Machine	4
	Tricep Press-Down	4
	Bicep Machine	4
	Bicep Machine Downset	1 x 25
3	Stiff Leg Deadlift*	4
	Stiff Leg Deadlift Downset	1 x 25
	Bent Row	4
	Seat Row	4
	Shrug	4
	Front Lat Pull	4
	Tricep Press Down	4
Week	Number of Reps	
1 and 2	8	
3 and 4	10	
5 and 6	15	
7 and 8	20	

*Performed with knees slightly bent, with two 45-pound plates.

Soccer Instructions

1. Always see a doctor, have a physical examination, and let him know your intentions and the type of exercise you plan on doing.
2. Start a new exercise program with moderation and build up through the program slowly.
3. This program is designed as an eight-week program, but can be extended for up to ten or twelve weeks by adding one week per weekly interval beginning with weeks one and two.
4. Use weights you can comfortably handle, performing slow and controlled positive movements. The negative movements should twice as slow as the positive ones.
5. Always stretch before and after your workout.
6. This program is three days per week with a minimum of one day of rest between each workout.
7. Downsets are always 25 percent less weight than performed on the main exercise.

TABLE 10-9

Running

Day	Exercise	Number of Sets
1 and 3	Squats or Leg Press	3
	Leg Extension	3
	Leg Curl	3
	Multi-Hip or Cable Crossover (front kick and back kick)	2
	Abductor or Cable Crossover (outer thigh pull)	2
	Adductor or Cable Crossover (inner thigh pull)	2
	Lunge	2
2	Chest or Bench Press	3
	Shoulder or Military Press	3
	Vertical Row	3
	Long Pull Machine	2
	Bicep Machine	3
	Tricep Machine	3
	Leg Curl	3
	Leg Raise	3
	Crunch	3

Week	Number of Reps (Distance)	Number of Reps (Sprinting)
1 and 2	25	10
3 and 4	30	12
5 and 6	40	15
7 and 8	60	20

Running Instructions

1. Always see a doctor, have a physical examination, and let him know your intentions and the type of exercise you plan on doing.
2. Start a new exercise program with moderation and build up through the program slowly.
3. This program is designed as an eight-week program, but can be extended for up to ten or twelve weeks by adding one week per weekly interval beginning with weeks one and two.
4. Use weights you can comfortably handle while performing slow and controlled positive movements. The negative movements should be twice as slow as the positive ones.
5. Always stretch before and after your workout.
6. This program may be utilized two to three days per week with a minimum of one day of rest between each workout.
7. When performing multi-hip and cable crossover exercises, the hips should never move or twist from side to side. Exercise is always performed in a slow and controlled fashion.

TABLE 10-10

Cycling

Day	Exercise	Number of Sets (x Extra Reps)	
1 and 3	Squat or Leg Press	3	
	Hack Squat	3	
	Leg Curl	3	
	Leg Extension	2	
	Standing Calf	2	
	Lunge with Weight	2	
	Lying-Down Scissor Kick	2	
2	Chest or Bench Press	2	
	Shoulder or Military Press	2	
	Bicep Curl	2	
	Bicep Machine	3	
	Tricep Machine	3	
	Leg Curl	3	
	Leg Raise	3 x 100 Distance	4 X 25 Sprinting
	Crunch	3 x 100 Distance	4 X 25 Sprinting

Week	Number of Reps (Distance)	Number of Reps (Sprinting)
1 and 2	25	10
3 and 4	35	12
5 and 6	45	15
7 and 8	50	20

Cycling Instructions

1. Always see a doctor, have a physical examination, and let him know your intentions and the type of exercise you plan on doing.
2. Start a new exercise program with moderation and build up through the program slowly.
3. This program is designed as an eight-week program, but can be extended for up to ten or twelve weeks by adding one week per weekly interval beginning with weeks one and two.
4. Use weights you can comfortably handle performing slow and controlled positive movements. The negative movements should twice as slow as the positive ones.
5. Always stretch before and after your workout.
6. This program is three days per week with a minimum of one day of rest between each workout.
7. When performing lunges with weight, never put weight on your shoulders, because of the risk of injury to the lower back. Hold the dumbbells in your hands and let them hang at your sides.

TABLE 10-11

Water & Snow Skiing

Day	Exercise	Number of Sets
1 and 3	Inner Thigh Pull	2
	Outer Thigh Pull	2
	Rear Kick	2
	Leg Press or Squat	2
	Leg Curl	2
	Leg Extension	2
	Front and Side Lunges	2
	Crunch	2
	Abdominal Machine	2
	Hanging Ab for Oblique (Side to Side)	2
2	Chest Press	3
	Shoulder Press	3
	Tricep Press-Downs	3
	Vertical Row Dips	3
	Front Lat Pull	3
	Lower Back Machine	3
	Bicep Curl	4
	Crunch	2
	Abdominal Machine	2
	Hanging Ab for Oblique (Side to Side)	2

Week	Number of Reps
1 and 4	15
5 and 7	20
8 and 12	25

Water & Snow Skiing

1. Always see a doctor, have a physical examination, and let him know your intentions and the type of exercise you plan on doing.
2. Start a new exercise program with moderation and build up through the program slowly.
3. This program is designed as a twelve-week program, but can be extended for up to fourteen or sixteen weeks by adding one week per weekly interval beginning with weeks one and four.
4. Use weights you can comfortably handle while performing slow and controlled positive movements. The negative movements should be twice as slow as the positive ones.
5. Always stretch before and after your workout.
6. This program is three days per week with a minimum of one day of rest between each workout. Legs are trained on day one and three. Chest is trained on day two.
7. When you do the inner/outer thigh pull and rear kick, your hips should never move or twist side to side. Exercise is always performed in a slow and controlled fashion.

TABLE 10-12

Swimming

Day	Exercise	Number of Sets	
1 and 3	Leg Curl	3	
	Leg Extension	3	
	Multi-Cable Crossover (front kick and back kick)	2	
	Lunges with Weight	2	
	Lying Scissor Kick	2	
2	Chest or Bench Presses	2	
	Pec Deck or Flies	2	
	Shoulder or Military Press	3	
	Front Raise	2	
	Rear Lateral Raise	2	
	Front Lateral Raise	2	
	Front Lat Pull	3	
	Bicep Machine	3	
	Tricep Machine	2	
	Low Back Machine	3	
	Long-Stroke Scissor Kick	2 x 5 Distance	2 X 20 Sprinting
	Leg Raise	2 x 5 Distance	2 X 20 Sprinting
	Crunch	2 x 5 Distance	2 X 20 Sprinting

Week	Number of Reps (Distance)	Number of Reps (Sprinting)
1 and 2	20	8
3 and 4	30	10
5 and 6	40	15
7 and 8	50	20

Swimming Instructions

1. Always see a doctor, have a physical examination, and let him know your intentions and the type of exercise you plan on doing.
2. Start a new exercise program with moderation and build up through the program slowly.
3. This program is designed as an eight-week program, but can be extended for up to ten or twelve weeks by adding one week per weekly interval beginning with weeks one and two.
4. Use weights you can comfortably handle while performing slow and controlled positive movements. The negative movements should twice as slow as the positive ones.
5. Always stretch before and after your workout.
6. This program should be done two to three days per week with a minimum of one day of rest between each workout.
7. Downsets are always 25 percent less weight than used on the main exercise.
8. For the long-stroke scissor kick, sit at the edge of a bench, round your back, and pull stomach in. Hold that position, straighten legs, and lift one foot toward the ceiling and the other foot toward the floor. Perform the full range of motion without bending the knees or twisting the hips. Do this in slow and controlled movements.

Twenty-one-year-old Mikhail Starov traveled halfway around the world from the Ukraine to train under John's guidance. Mike's success speaks for itself, when he set twelve World Records at the 1996 World Powerlifting Championship in New York City. In fourteen weeks, his body fat decreased from 32 percent to 14 percent while maintaining a body weight of 238 pounds. Mike increased his best competition squat from 733 pounds to 940 pounds, his best competition bench press from 460 pounds to 505 pounds, and his best competition deadlift from 740 pounds to 800 pounds. His best total was 1800 pounds. Mikhail now holds the record for the greatest total in the history of his country in any weight class—2245 pounds! When asked about his training, Mikhail said John is the best strength trainer he has ever seen, with knowledge of training, nutrition, and supplementation.

Mikhail Starov is pictured at the finish of the 940 pounds Junior World Record squat.

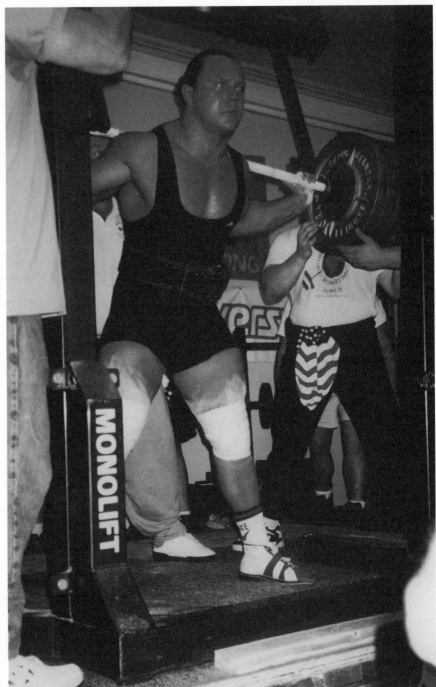

Chapter Eleven

Powerlifting

Many people will probably purchase this book just to read this particular section because of the success I've had creating world-champion lifters. So here it is from one of the top strength coaches in the world, an outline of the Schaeffer and Clark strength systems approach, what I consider the steps to building a champion.

Step 1
A Body Composition Test

This is very important. First you need to establish your body fat percentage, and then strive to attain a preferred 12 to 14 percent for male lifters and 13 to 15 percent for female lifters. Obviously, the more lean mass you have to work with, the greater the potential for big lifts. You should be careful not to go below the recommended percentages of body fat or you may increase the possibility of injury by being too lean. This is a condition in which the muscles' natural cushion for handling heavy weights is decreased.

Step 2
Design a Nutrition Program

Designing a nutrition program will help decrease your body fat and increase your lean mass, or stabilize your lean mass under intense training. In order to reach your goal, start with 0.8 grams of protein per each pound of lean mass. For example, consume 20 to 25 grams of protein per serving every two-and-a-half to three hours, and a 30-gram protein serving along with a small portion of carbohydrates within fifteen minutes after training. Adjust your carbohydrates and fats to support your energy expenditures. Monitor lean mass gains and adjust your protein percentages to increase or decrease accordingly. (See Food Intake list, page 86.)

Step 3
Design a Supplement Program

This must suit your needs. The following is an example of a typical program:

- Take two to three aminos at mid-morning, mid-afternoon, and at bedtime.
- Take egg or whey protein within fifteen minutes after workout.
- For a low-intensity workout, have one serving of creatine supplement a day. For a medium-intensity workout, have two servings a day. A high-intensity workout requires three servings a day.
- Take one ounce of colloidal mineral drink in the morning and one ounce in the evening.

- Drink water before your workout, drinking slowly one hour prior to training. Drink five to six ounces of water every fifteen minutes during training.
- Consume energy source carbohydrates and herb formulas thirty to sixty minutes prior to training.
- Use all supplements according to manufacturer's directions.

Step 4
Videotape Your Workout

Do some videotaping of your sessions, making sure to include at least one of each of the following: dead lift, squat, and bench. This will help check bio-mechanics, leverage, and technique so you may make adjustments accordingly.

Step 5
Lay Out a Three-Week Cross-Fiber Training Schedule

Using white, intermediate, and red fibers for increased lean mass and body-fat loss, which will build the upper end of your anaerobic threshold for more effective recovery between lifts. (See Table 11-2.)

Step 6
Establish Equipment Needs

This includes shirts, suits, shoes, belts, etc.

Protein Need Factor Chart

You will need the following amount of protein per day per pound of lean body mass.

.5g	Sedentary—non-active
.6g	Light fitness exercise
.7g	Moderate exercise—three times per week
.8g	Daily training—some weight and aerobics
.9g	Heavy weight training
1.0g	Heavy weight training plus sports activity four to seven times weekly

Step 7
Establish an Eight- to Ten-Week Four-Day Explosive Program

Using a combination of the muscle overload theory and neurological activity training, it is possible to capitalize on strength gains. (See Table 11-3.)

Step 8
Establish an Actual Power Program

Wear protective gear during the power phase. For the first four to five weeks, wear shirts and suits bigger than the ones you will use in competition. For the last two to three weeks, use competition equipment. Remember, few strength gains are made in an actual power phase. You are only maximizing your potential from your pre-training programs. Never underemphasize the importance of your pre-power training. This includes all aspects from your workout programs to nutrition and supplementation.

TABLE 11-1

Sample Supplementation Program

Time	Supplement	Suggested Serving
6:30 A.M.	Colloidal mineral drink	1 oz.—best taken on an empty stomach
7:30 A.M.	1 Serving of Creatine*	Creatine serving 8 oz. water First meal 8 oz. water
9:00 A.M.	2 aminos	Second meal 8 oz. Water Take aminos with grape juice 8 oz. Water
12:30 P.M.	1 Serving of Creatine*	Creatine serving 8 oz. water Third meal Pre-workout carbohydrate herb drink
3:30 P.M.	2 aminos	Fourth meal 8 oz. water Aminos with orange juice 8 oz. water
6:30 P.M.	1 Serving of Creatine*	Creatine serving 8 oz water Fifth meal 1 oz. colloidal mineral drink
11:00 P.M.	2 aminos	Aminos with grape Juice—best taken on an empty stomach

*Adjust your creatine intake according to the intensity of your training. During low-intensity training, take it only at 7:30 A.M. Take creatine at 7:30 A.M. and 6:30 P.M. during medium-intensity training. High-intensity training allows creatine at 7:30 A.M., 12:30 P.M., and 6:30 P.M.

Step 9
Establish Pre-Contest Nutritional Needs

Do this for two days before the contest and on the day it takes place. During the preceding two days, you need a ratio of twenty-five percent protein to fifty-five percent carbs to twenty percent fat. You should drink eight to ten glasses of water both days, drinking slowly. On the day of the contest, eat a breakfast consisting of two egg whites in a whole wheat bread sandwich, one bowl of oatmeal, and a half slice of cantaloupe.

If you are competing in the afternoon, eat a bowl of oatmeal and about ten grams of protein every three hours until one and a half hours before the contest. During the contest, eat one wedge of apple (one inch wide) and drink three to five ounces of water every fifteen to twenty minutes.

Typical Food Intake For Fat Loss & Lean Mass Increase

Monday, Wednesday, and Friday

7:00 to 8 A.M.
1 cup oatmeal
1 egg white
1 slice lite bread
1 slice cantaloupe
(4 aminos)

10:00 to 10:30 A.M.
1 baked potato
1 slice cantaloupe

12:00 to 12:30 P.M.
1 chicken breast
½ cup rice
1 baked potato

10:00 to 12:30 P.M.
3 aminos

2:30 to 3:00 P.M.
1 chicken breast
Orange (juice)

5:30 to 6:00 P.M.
½ cup pasta salad
Veggies
Salad
1 baked potato
(4 aminos)

Tuesday, Thursday, and Saturday

7:00 to 8:00 A.M.
1 bowl bran cereal
1 slice cantaloupe
(4 aminos)

10:00 to 10:30 A.M.
1 slice lite bread
1 slice cantaloupe

12:00 to 12:30 P.M.
½ cup pasta

1 chicken breast
Salad
(3 aminos)

1:00 to 2:00 P.M.
½ cup rice
Broccoli

5:00 to 6:00 P.M.
2 chicken breasts
1 cup rice
Veggies
Salad
(4 aminos)

Sunday

7:00 to 8 A.M.
1 cup oatmeal
1 slice lite bread
1 slice cantaloupe
2 egg whites
(4 aminos)

12:00 to 12:30 P.M.
1 chicken breast
½ cup Rice
1 baked potato
(3 aminos)

5:00 to 6:00 P.M.
½ cup pasta
Salad
1 baked potato
Veggies
(4 aminos)

Necessary Snacks Between Meals
Fruit
Popcorn with no butter or salt
Low-fat, sugar-free yogurt
Rice Cakes

Liquids
Water
Juice

TABLE 11-2

Endurance Program

Day	Exercise
1	Squat or Leg Press
	Butt-buster
	Leg Curl
	Leg Extension
	Abductor
	Adductor
	Calf
	Leg Raise
	Crunch Twist
	Crunches
	Rotary Torso
2	Chest Press
	Pec Deck
	Shoulder Press
	Upright Row
	Pull-ups
	Low Back
	Bicep Curl
	Tricep Extension
	Leg Raise
	Crunch Twist
	Crunches
	Rotary Torso
3	Stiff Deadlift From Bottom of Knee
	Bent Row
	Vertical Row
	Front Lat Pull
	Trap Shrug
	Leg Raise
	Crunch Twist
	Crunches
	Rotary Torso

Week	Number of Reps	Number of Sets
1	10 Very Slow (3.5 Sec. Positive & 3.5 sec. Negative) 10 Explosive	2
2	10 Very Slow (3.5 Sec. Positive & 3.5 sec. Negative) 15 Explosive	2
3	15 Very Slow (3.5 Sec. Positive & 3.5 sec. Negative) 15 Explosive	1

NOTE: Slow movements are followed immediately by explosive movements with no rest in between.

TABLE 11-3

Four-Day Explosive White Fiber Program

Day	Exercise	Number of Sets
1	Bench Press	3
	Camber Bench Press	2
	Reverse Bench Press	2
	Shoulder Press	2
	French Curl	3
	Tricep Machine	2
	Tricep Push Down	2
2	Squat	3
	Leg Press	2
	Hack Squat	2
	Leg Extension	2
	Leg Curl	3
	Standing Calf	2
	Seated Calf	2
	Plus any three of the following:	
	Bar Curls of Choice	2
	Bicep Machine	2
	Dumbbell Curl	2
	Concentration Curl	2
3	Incline Bench Press	3
	Decline Bench Press	2
	Military Press	2
	Lateral Raise	2
	Any two Tricep Exercises	2
4	Stiff Leg Deadlift	3
	Bent Row	2
	One-Arm Dumbbell Row	2
	Vertical or Seat Row	2
	Camber Bar Trap Shrug	2
	Front Lat Pull	2
	Any two Bicep Exercises	2

Week	Reps
1–3	10 Explosive
4–7	12 Explosive
8–10	15 Explosive

Work your abdominals two to three days a week, up to twelve sets. Make sure you understand the difference between explosive and ballistic lifts. Explosive lifts start slowly and accelerate through the lift. Never bounce your lifts ballistically. You should be lifting 45 to 55 percent of your maximum weight during these exercises.

Sample Power Program

Week	Sets	Reps	Squat	Bench	Deadlift
1	1	15	230	260	250
2	1	10	260	275	280
3	1	8	290	290	450
4	1	6	320	305	300
5	1	4	350	320	500
6	1	3	380	335	350
7	1	2	510	350	540
8	1	2	540	365	None
9	Contest	Contest	Contest	Contest	Contest

The above sets and the following assistance do not include warm-up sets. On overloads always stay in the safety of racks and have adequate spotters. Extreme care must be taken when doing overloads.

TABLE 11-5

Assistance Work

Day	Exercise	Number of Sets	Number of Reps
1 Squat Day (100–150 over a maximum of 750)*			
	Stand Up	1	10
	Leg Press	5	3
	Leg Curl	2	15
	Standing Calf	2	15
2 Bench Day (100–150 over a maximum of 550	1 x 10 sec. only)**		
	Camber Bar	5	3
	Tricep Push Down	2	15
	Military Press	2	15
	Bicep Bar Curl	2	15
	Hammer Curl	2	15
3 Deadlift Day			
	Rack Pull 750***	5	1
	Bent Row	2	15
	Shrug	2	15
	Front Lat Pull	2	15
4 Light Bench Day			
	Close Grip Bench Press	5	3
	Reverse Bench Press	2	15
	Incline Bench Press	2	15
	Bicep Curl	2	15

 * Hold at top for ten seconds in a standing position, only moving bar two or three inches. Do not walk out of racks (use a spotter).

 ** Do not take bar out of racks. Move toward the upright until your head is off the bench and you can hold bar in locked position without coming out of racks (use a spotter).

 *** Pull from mid-Knee.

TABLE 11-6

Sample of Maximum Lifts

Lift	Squat	Bench	Deadlift	Total
1	540	365	540	1445
2	570	380	570	1520
3	600	400	600	1600

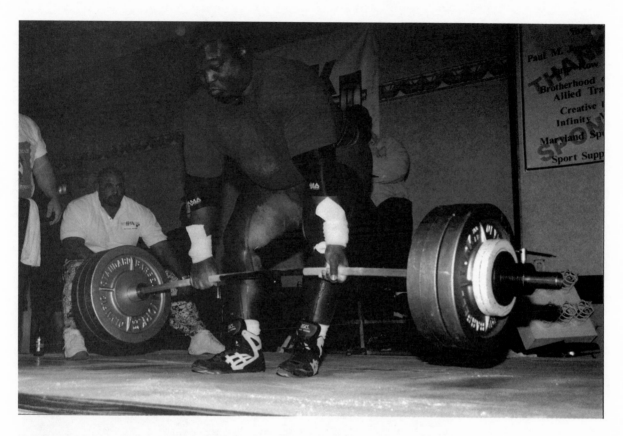

Jr. Hunt is a multi-World Champion and one of the strongest people at a body weight of 400 plus pounds. Jr. attributes a big part of his success to John's training and nutrition concepts.

The parents of sixteen-year-old John Richardson and fifteen-year-old Andrew High realized the importance of seeking out a trainer skilled in working with young athletes. After nine weeks of proper nutritional supplementation, diet, and exercise, each athlete increased his lean muscle weight by fifteen pounds and almost doubled his physical strength levels. Their high school coaches were amazed at their tremendous progress in this short period of time.

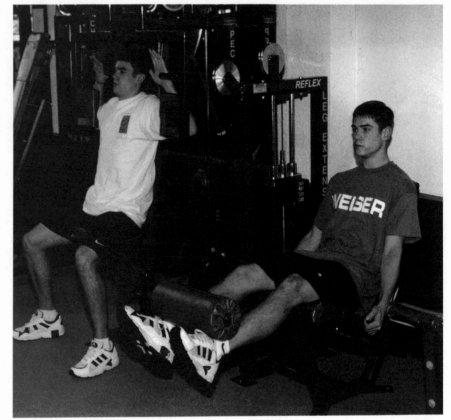

Chapter Twelve

Weight Training for Youth

In my role as a fitness trainer and as a coach, I've often had people ask me for advice on how young people can best participate in weight training. The guidelines I follow for answering these questions are very conservative. The reason for this is that one of the most radical differences between youthful and adult physiology is at issue here: bone composition. Bones and the leverage they provide are at the very heart of weight lifting.

The skeleton of an infant is unique in two ways. First, it contains a very high percentage of external cartilage, and second, unlike adult bones, the insides of babies' bones are entirely cartilage. The adult skeleton's external cartilage is pretty much confined to joints and junctures, and all cartilage that was once inside their bones has been replaced with a mostly hardened combination of compact bone and bone with lots of spaces in it filled with marrow, called spongy bone. The degree of softness, or cartilaginous flexibility, in the bones of any young person who has yet to reach full growth falls somewhere on a gradient between those of a soft infant and those of a hardened, fully grown adult.

The closer a person is to the infant beginning of this gradient, the more they should be kept from doing any weight training at all. As they come closer to the adult conclusion of it

they can probably do some weight lifting without risk of injury. However, the training still has to be modified carefully since being almost an adult in this case does not mean that you are as safe from injury as an adult would be. The reason for this is that the last place where bone cartilage hardens is near the end of the long bones, where for a time it forms a border between the shank of the bone and the epiphysis process. These are the knobby ends of the long bones, which have to carry the compression and thrust of the major body joints, like the hip and the knee. Submitting these still flexible impact points to repetitious, high-stress movements risks injuring them and disrupting normal growth.

Teenagers, we don't need to be reminded, have a lot of concerns about how they look, and they can be a lot of fun to coach, because weight training is just great for helping out with this problem. On the other hand, another teenage virtue, enthusiasm, has to be watched for here. Young people in weight training should have careful, skilled supervision. I also might mention that a lot of young people who want to work out but still have substantial time to put in before their bones stop growing can be steered toward gymnastics, a great conditioning activity that provides good use for all that cartilage that kids have, as you may have noticed while watching the Olympics.

Following is a list of my suggestions for putting together a safe weight training program for youth.

- Check the psychological state of the young person as well as the physical to see if he or she is disciplined and careful enough to do the program.
- Make sure the training occurs in a highly supervised environment.
- Avoid free weights. Use selectorized machines instead to minimize the risk of injury.
- Never perform exercise with overload weight techniques. To aid in the development of flexibility, use a full range of motion on all exercises.
- Don't train for competition, or to reach peaks in general.
- Always warm up before weight training and cool down afterward.
- Combining weight training with the pursuit of another sport like swimming or track works well for young people.
- Avoid nutritional supplementation, except, of course, those recommended by a physician. Try to make sure that some rules for a complete balanced diet are being followed.

- We recommend training with weights two to three times a week.
- Make certain the young person is thoroughly coached in technique before they lift any weight.
- To learn proper technique, use repetitions of fifteen in two to three sets. Practice high reps with low weight in general.
- To increase resistance loads, drop back to six to eight reps and increase the weight by two to five pounds until sets of fifteen are again achieved.
- Sessions should not exceed forty minutes.
- Never do maximum single lifts or any type of overload training.

Reviewing this chapter and its guidelines should help illustrate that there is no easy way to tell the best age at which to start a child on a weight training program. Proper assessments must be made and strict guidelines must be followed to prevent risk of injury. Always use extreme caution and consideration in developing a weight training program for youth. Obtain assistance from a qualified youth instructor whenever possible. Care and caution are the keys . . . with care and caution, supervised weight training can benefit young people too.

Chapter Thirteen

Exercise Instructions

Leg Exercises

The following foot positions are used for calf work.

1. With toes pointing in, you work the outer calf muscle.
2. With toes pointing out, you work the inner calf muscle.
3. With toes straight, you work the center calf muscle.

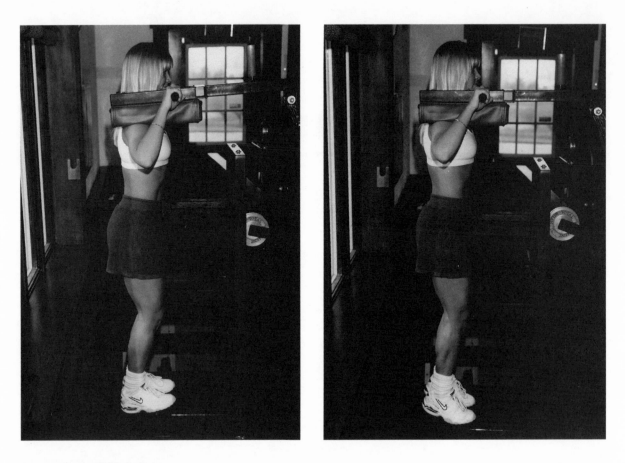

Standing Calf Raises

- Use either a barbell on your shoulders with a block of wood to stand on or a standing calf machine.
- Stand on the block with your heels extended into space.
- Keep your knees slightly bent and your back straight throughout the exercise.
- Push up on your toes, then lower your heels toward the floor, feeling the calf muscles stretch.
- Starting from a low position of movement, come up on your toes as far as possible.

Leg Exercises

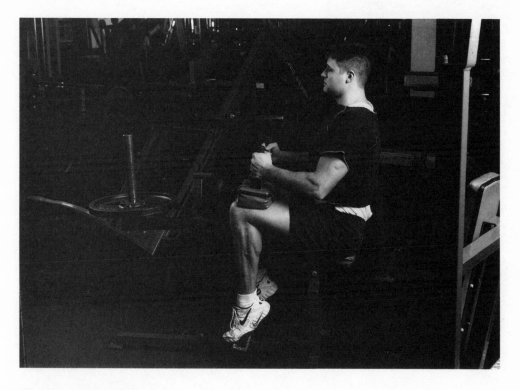

Seated Calf Raises

- Sit at the machine with your toes on the block and your knees hooked under the crossbar.
- Keep the weight just above your knees on the thighs.
- Slowly lower your heels toward the floor, testing the stretch to be sure it stays in the comfort zone.
- Push up on your toes to full extension.
- Do not rock back and forth while going through the movements of the exercise.

Leg Exercises

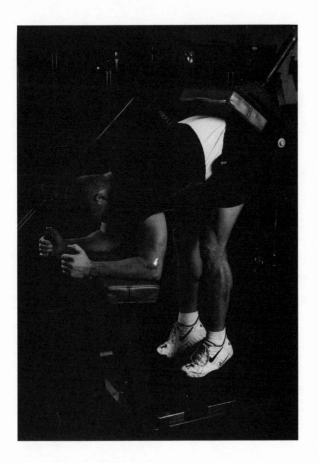

Donkey Calf Raises

- Use a block of wood to stand on and a bench to lean on if a machine is not available. Without a machine, you will need a partner to sit across your hips.
- Bend at the waist and place your weight well back on your hips to keep pressure away from the lower back.
- Stand on the balls of your feet.
- Holding your knees steady in a slightly bent position, lower your heels toward the floor for a full stretch.
- Use a full range of motion, coming back up on your toes and flexing calves at the top.

Leg Exercises

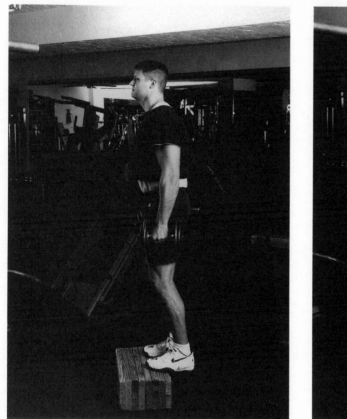 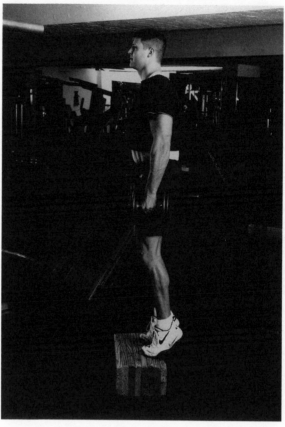

Free-Standing Toe Raises with Dumbbells

- Use a block of wood to stand on.
- Stand upright, holding a dumbbell in each hand.
- Stand on the balls of your feet with your heels extended into space.
- Keeping your knees steady in a slightly bent position, lower your heels toward the floor for a full stretch.
- Use a full range of motion coming back up, flexing the calves as you stand on the balls of your feet.

Leg Exercises

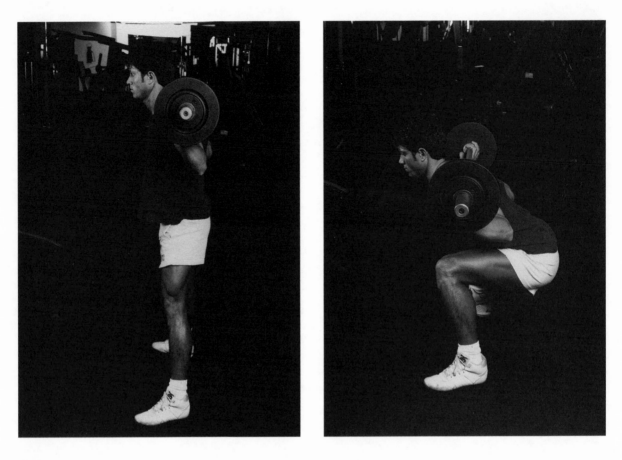

Squats

When doing squats, varying the position of your feet will target different areas of the leg muscles. A wide stance works the inside of the thighs and the hips. A close stance works the outside of the thighs. The basic stance for squats places your feet shoulder width apart, your toes slightly out.

- Position the barbell well back on the shoulders, below and off your neck.
- Keep your head and chest up and your back straight.
- When you reach the down position, your thighs should be parallel, or slightly below parallel, to the floor.
- Thrust back with your hips, as though sitting in a chair, to keep knees from bending out too far.
- Do not bounce. Use the muscles of your thighs and hips, not the back muscles, to return to an upright position. Keep your feet flat on the platform and don't lock your knees.

Leg Exercises

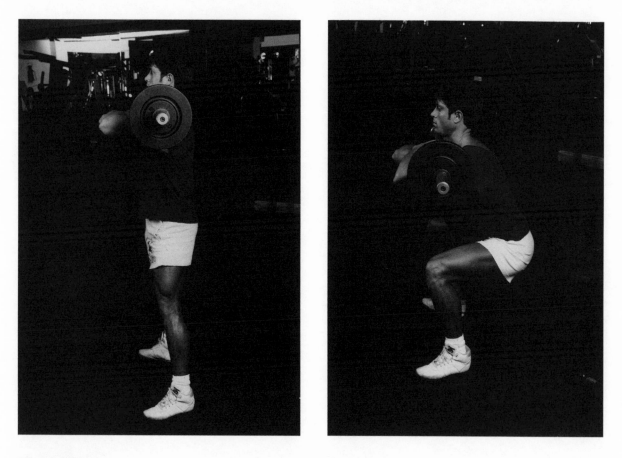

Front Squats

- Cross your arms while keeping the elbows high, and grasp the bar with both hands.
- The barbell should rest in front of the deltoid muscles as you hold it.
- Bend your knees, keeping your head and chest up and your back straight.
- Lower yourself until your thighs are parallel to the floor and sit back on your hips.
- Push up slowly, keeping your back straight.

Leg Exercises

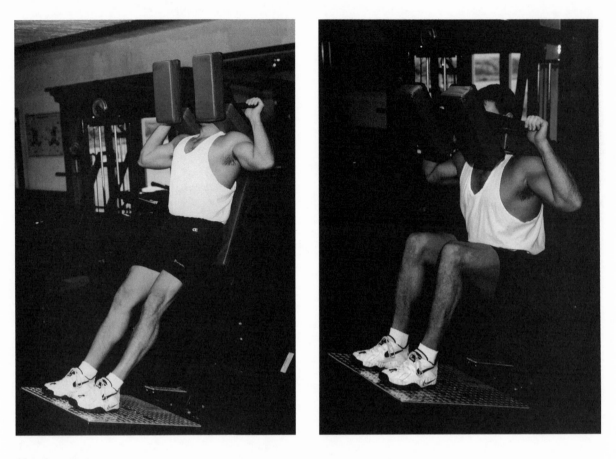

Hack squats

- Keep your head up and your back straight against the machine pad as you place your shoulders under the pads.
- Keep your feet flat on the platform, six inches apart, your toes straight and your knees in line with your toes.
- Lower yourself all the way down, bending your knees at a sharp angle.
- Keeping constant tension on the leg muscles, push strongly from the heels of your feet, driving the weight up until your legs are fully extended.

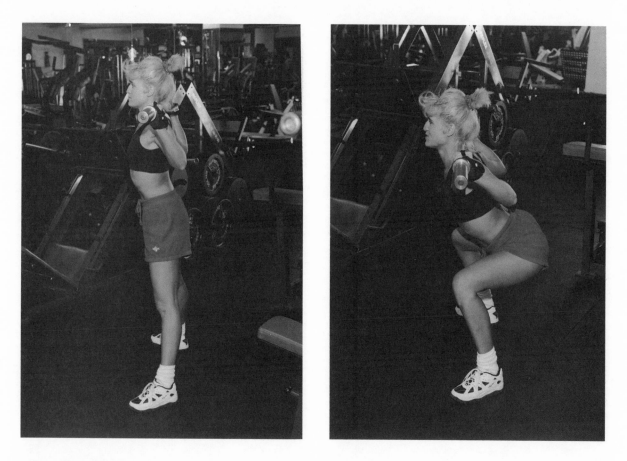

High Bar Squats

- Grip the bar with the placement of your hands slightly wider than shoulder width.
- Rest the bar on your rear deltoid muscles, very high on the back of your neck.
- Keep your head and chest up and your back straight as you bend your knees and lower yourself.
- Sit back on your hips with your thighs parallel to the floor before returning slowly to a standing position.

Leg Exercises

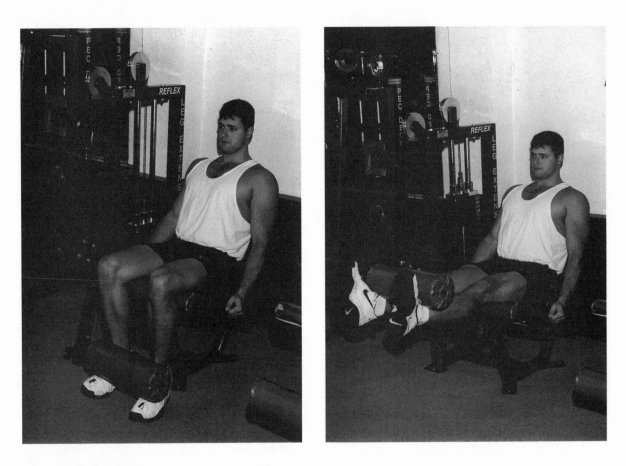

Leg Extensions

- Sitting in a leg extension machine, press your back against the pad and the back of your knees against the edge of the seat as you hook your feet under the padded bar.
- Keep your toes in line with your knees as you fully extend legs until they are parallel to the floor. Do not lock your knees.
- Contract the quadriceps muscles at the front of your thighs, then lower the weight slowly until your feet are farther back than your knees.
- Don't lift yourself off the seat while lifting with your legs.

Leg Exercises

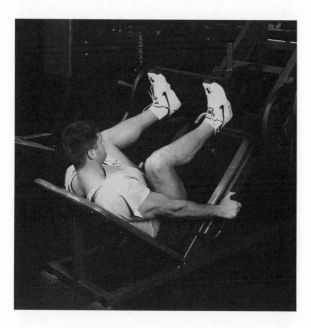

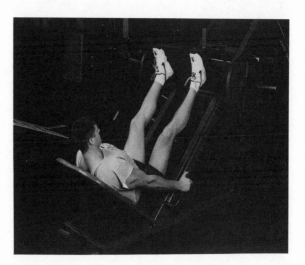

Leg Presses

- Position yourself in a leg press machine with your back flat against the upright seat and your legs extended.
- Grasp the handles or the seat edge for stability as you control the weight's descent by bending your knees. Do not push back with your legs.
- Bring your knees down on either side of your chest, toward your shoulders. Do not hit your chest.
- Keep your hips down; don't tilt your pelvis.
- Keep your feet flat against the foot platform. Push from your heels and return the legs to an extended position without locking your knees.

Leg Exercises

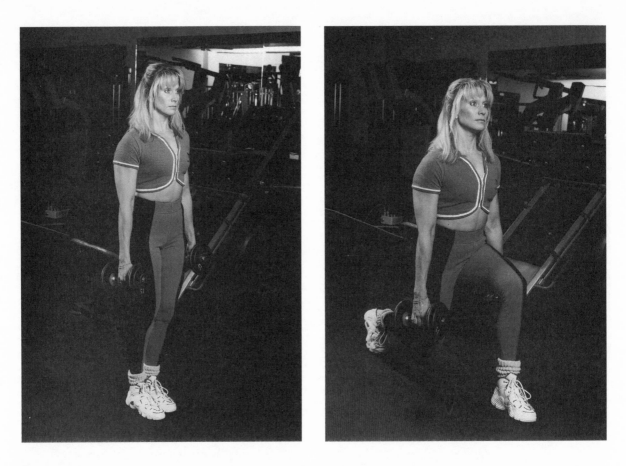

Lunges

- Take dumbbells in each hand while keeping your head forward, your back straight, and your feet together.
- Step forward far enough so the thigh of the stepping leg is parallel with the floor and your trailing knee is almost touching the floor.
- With one decisive movement of the stepping leg, return to the original position and step out with the other leg.
- You can also do all your repetitions with one leg, then switch and repeat for the other.

Leg Exercises

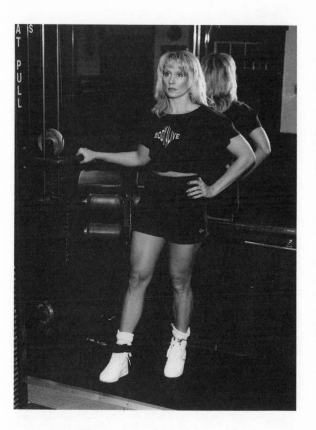
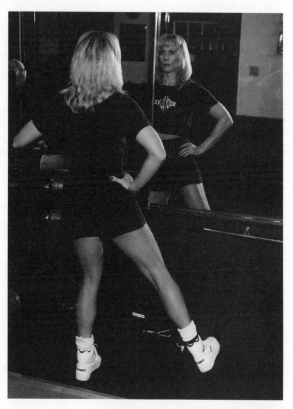

Cable Pulls

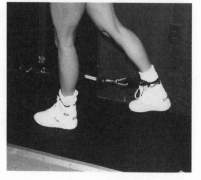

- Stand straight during the exercise, using the machine or stationary bar for support.
- Keep your hips straight, head forward.
- Inner pull: approaching the machine from the side, attach the ankle strap to your leg closest to the machine. In the exercise movement, pull your leg across your body, leading with the heel.
- Outer pull: approaching the machine from the side, attach the ankle strap to the leg farthest from the machine. During the exercise, pull your leg out and away from your body, driving the heel toward the ceiling.
- Pull to the rear: face the machine and attach the ankle strap to your leg. Kick straight back, keeping your foot flexed upward.
- Alternate legs.

Leg Exercises

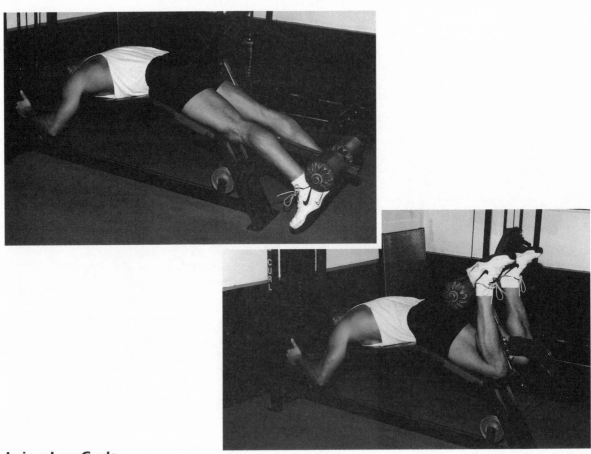

Lying Leg Curls

- Lie facedown on the machine. Keep your stomach against the pad and the back of your heels under the rollers.
- Keep your toes in line with your knees and your feet flexed.
- Contract your hamstrings, lifting your heels against the resistance until your calves are at right angles to your thighs.
- Release the contraction slowly, lowering your legs back to the starting position.
- Hold on to the handles or the edge of the seat to keep yourself from lifting off the bench.

Leg Exercises

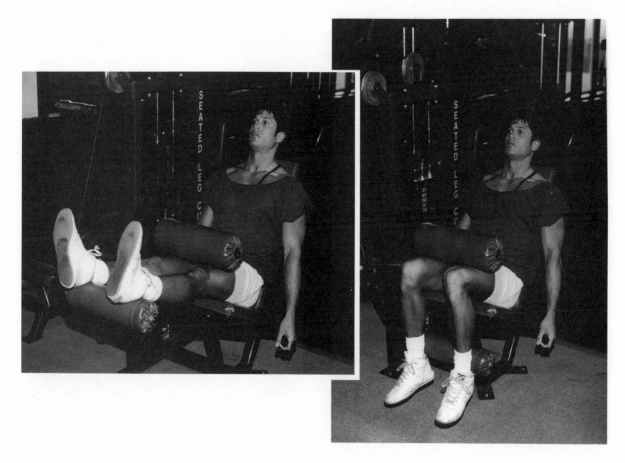

Seated Leg Curls

- Seated in the machine, press the lower part of your back against the back pad of the seat.
- With legs extended and feet flexed, pull the roller pad down, pulling your heels toward your buttocks until your knees are at a 90-degree angle.
- Release slowly.

Leg Exercises

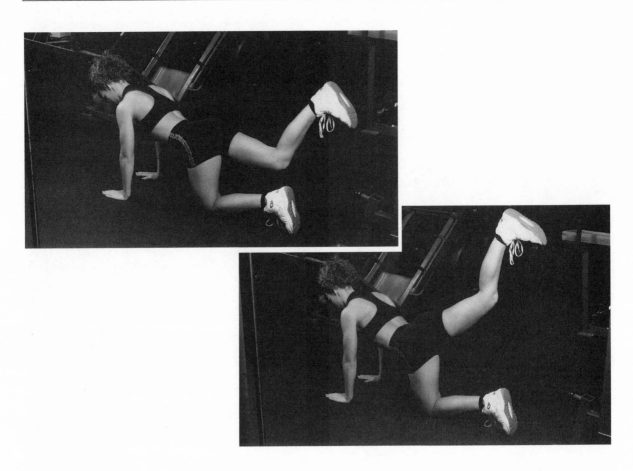

Butt-busters

- Get on all fours, elbow and knee position, with the knee you are not using slightly ahead.
- Leading with your heel, push your leg up and away from the body to a 45-degree angle, or as far as you can.
- On return, the negative side of the lift, do not let your knee drop below the level of your spine. Keep your back straight.

Leg Exercises

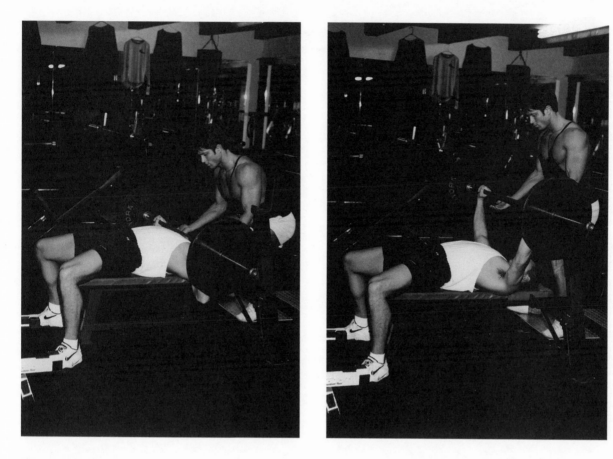

Bench Press

- Lie with your hips on the bench, your legs off the end, and your feet flat on the floor.
- Position your hands carefully on the bar so that as you lower it to your chest your hands are far enough apart that your forearms point straight up, perpendicular to the floor. This is usually slightly wider than shoulder width.
- Lower weight to the mid-pectoral area, across nipples.
- After coming to a complete stop, press the bar upward until the arms can be locked.
- Move slowly and under control; do not bounce the bar off your chest. Do not arch your back.

Chest Exercises

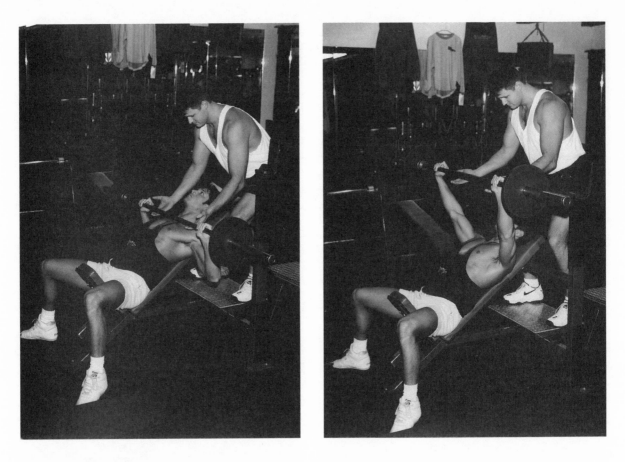

Incline Bench Press

- Lie on the incline bench with your hips on the seat and your feet flat on the floor.
- Take the bar with your hands placed slightly wider than shoulder width apart. See the bench press exercise for positioning hands.
- Lower the bar to your upper chest, just below your chin.
- Keep your elbows back until you feel a full stretch as you lower the bar.
- After you come to a stop, push the bar up and slightly away from your face at a 45-degree angle.
- Do not let the bar drift forward as you push up. Do not arch your back.

Chest Exercises

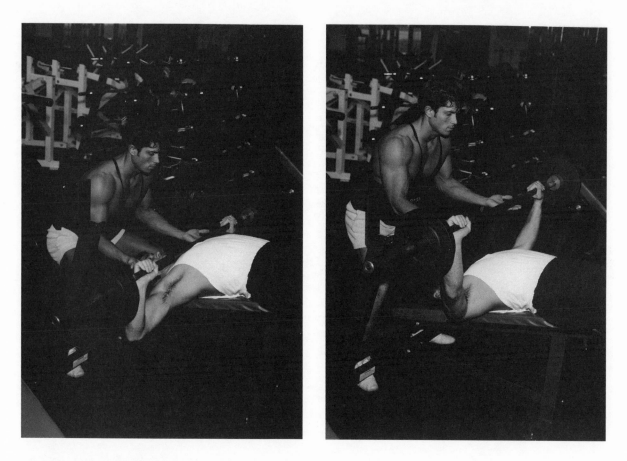

Decline Bench Press

- Position your hands as in the bench press exercise.
- Bring the bar down to your lower pectoral area.
- Press the bar upward and slightly away from your face. Do not bounce.

Chest Exercises

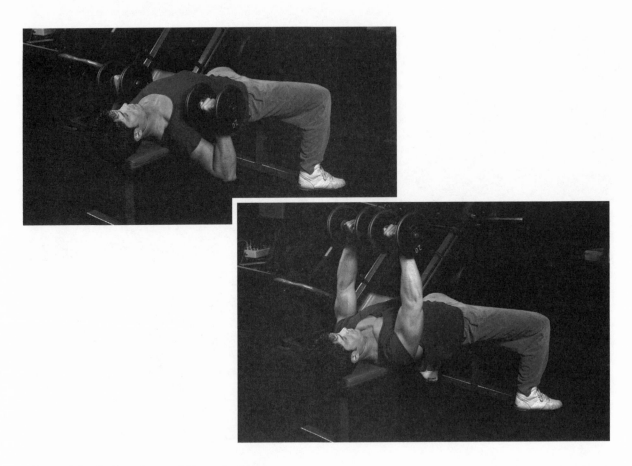

Dumbbell Cambered Bench Press

- The exercise can be done flat, on an incline, or on a decline.
- Position the dumbbell on either side of the chest, as if using a bar.
- Drive the dumbbells up as if using a bar, then stretch down slowly back to the starting position.

Chest Exercises

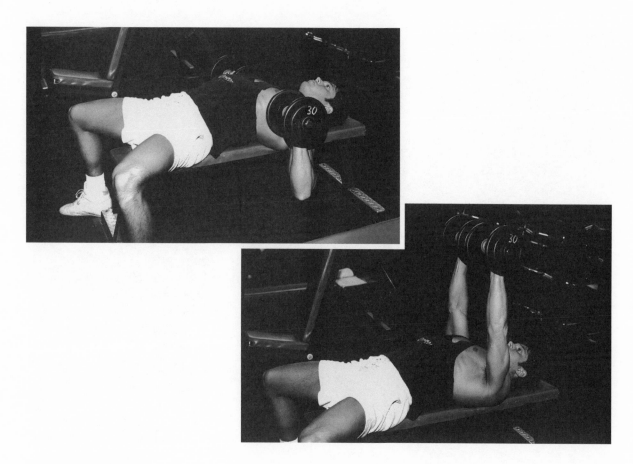

Dumbbell Press

- The exercise can be done flat, on an incline, or on a decline.
- Position the dumbbell on either side of the chest as if using a bar.
- Drive the dumbbells up as if using a bar, then stretch back down to the starting position.

Chest Exercises

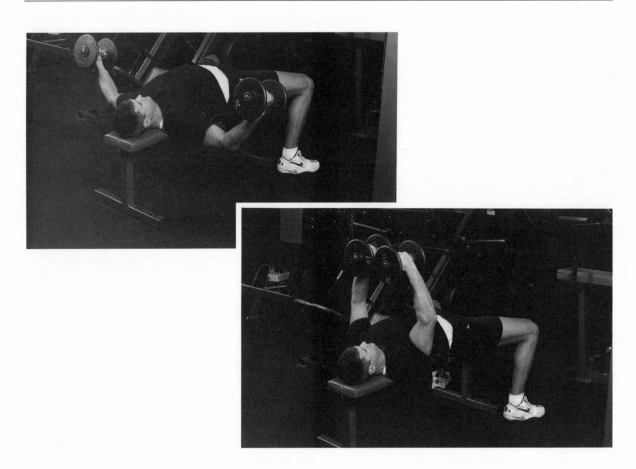

Dumbbell Flies

- The exercise can be done flat, on an incline, or on a decline.
- Lie on a bench, holding the dumbbells at arm's length above you, with your palms facing and your elbows slightly bent.
- Open your arms, lowering weights out and down to either side, while keeping your arms slightly bent.
- Bring the weights to a stop when you have given the pectoral muscles a good stretch.
- Lift the weights back up in the same wide arc, as though reaching around a tree.

Chest Exercises

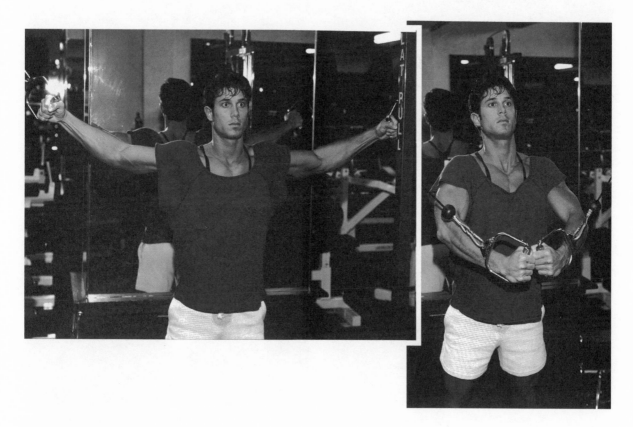

Cable Crossovers

- The exercise can be done with upper or lower pulleys.
- With your feet shoulder width apart, grasp the pulley handle in each hand.
- Take a position of leaning forward slightly and hold it throughout the exercise.
- As you lean forward, allow your arms to extend out to either side, with your elbows slightly bent.
- Next, draw your hands down and toward each other, thoroughly contracting the pectoral muscles.
- Finish by bringing your arms and elbows back to shoulder height.

Chest Exercises

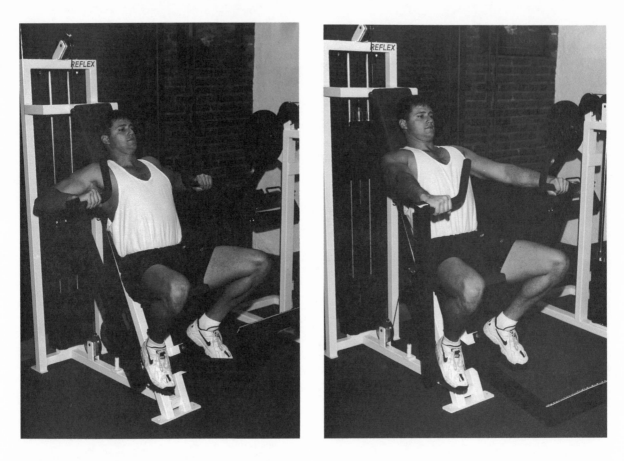

Chest Press Machine

- Position the seat so that your hands can be placed on the lifting bar at chest level.
- Position your hands so that the hands and elbows remain in line during the lift.
- Press forward and up on the bar until your arms lock.
- Come back down slowly to the starting position.
- The press machine makes movements in the exercise very regular and predictable. It is especially helpful if you are injured or do not want to risk lifting a free weight.

Chest Exercises

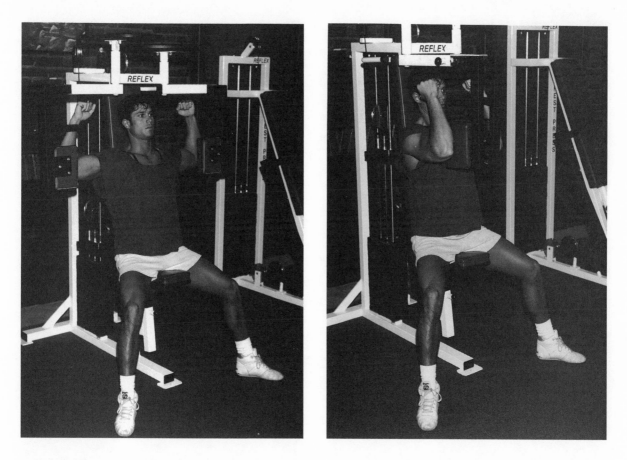

Pec Deck

- Position your elbows on pads of the machine so your arms are parallel.
- Pull your elbows together while contracting your pectorals.
- Slowly separate, opening your elbows back to the starting point.
- Be sure to drive with your elbows, not your hands.

Chest Exercises

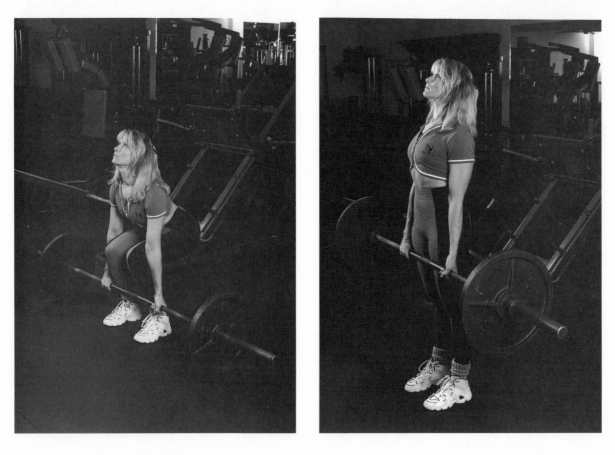

Conventional Deadlift

- Place a barbell on the floor in front of you and position your feet six to eight inches apart, pointing away from each other at 45 degrees.
- Grip the bar outside of your legs, keeping your head up and back straight, with one hand over the other.
- Sit back on your hips, keeping the bar against your shins with your chin pointed toward the ceiling.
- Lift the bar, holding it against your body until your body is fully upright; throw your chest out and shoulders back.
- Bend the knees and keep the back straight as you lower the weight to the floor.
- Keeping the chin up and the back straight is very important both to protect the lower back from injury and to mobilize the largest number of muscle groups possible for the lift.

Back Exercises

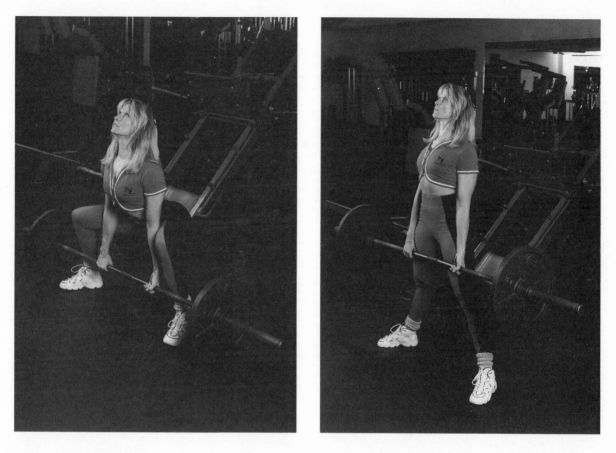

Sumo Deadlift

- Place your feet two to three inches wider than your shoulders, pointing away from each other at about 45 degrees, as you stand in front of the barbell resting on the floor.
- Position your hands on the bar inside your legs, but without restricting your ability to expand your chest.
- Sit back on your hips to mobilize your leg muscles fully for the lift.
- Continue the pull until your body is fully erect.
- Bend your knees and bend over to lower the weight.
- This deadlift method emphasizes hip and leg strength over back strength.

Back Exercises

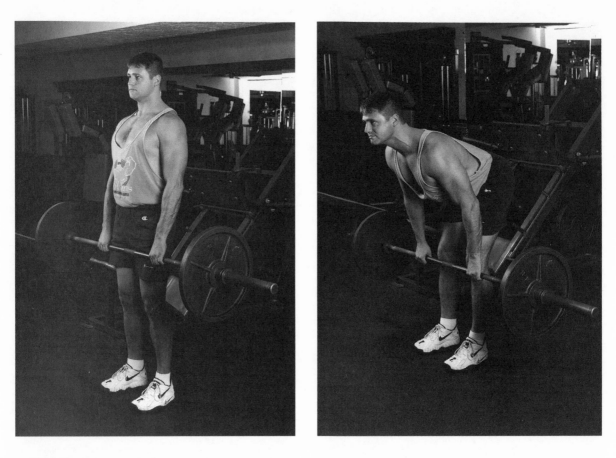

Stiff-legged Deadlift

- To perform the lifting half of this exercise, use the steps given above for conventional deadlift, except that you only allow your legs to bend slightly.
- Once you start to bend from your upright position back toward the floor, keep your head and chest up and your back slightly arched. Keep the bar against your legs.
- Bring the bar down to just below your knees, giving a good stretch to your hamstrings.
- Return to upright position.
- Stand on a block or on two 45-pound plates to increase the stretch to the floor.

Back Exercises

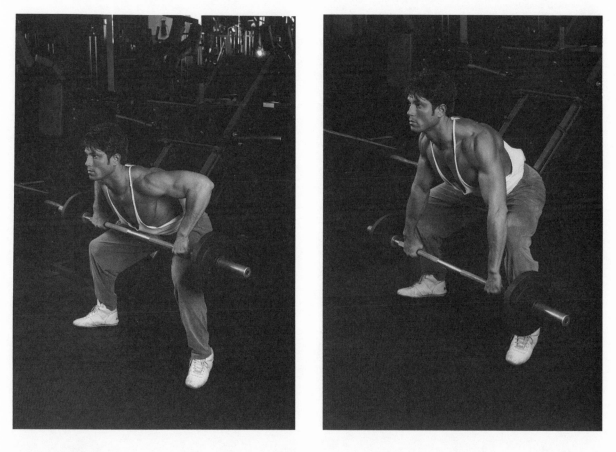

Barbell Rows

- Standing with your feet a few inches apart, bend over and grasp the barbell with an overhand grip slightly wider than shoulder width.
- Remaining bent over with your knees bent, bring the barbell off the floor, but no farther up than the point where your upper torso becomes parallel with the floor.
- Starting with the bar hanging at arm's length, nearly touching your shinbone, use the muscles in the middle and upper back to pull the weight up toward the upper abdominal area.
- Lower the weight under control back to the hanging position below you, ready for the next rep.
- Concentrate on working the back muscles in this exercise, not letting the arms take over.

Back Exercises

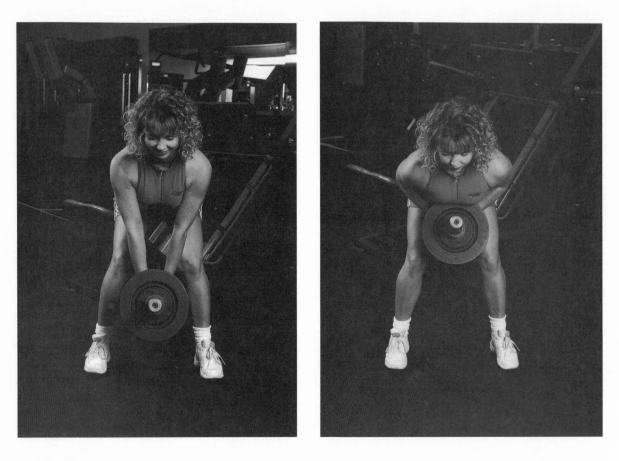

T-Bar Rows

- With your knees slightly bent, bend down and use an overhand grip to grasp the handles of the T-bar machine.
- Keeping your back straight and your head up, lift the bar until your body is at a 45-degree angle. Staying at this angle, continue lifting the bar to touch your chest.
- Lower the weight slowly to arm's length without touching the floor if you are doing reps.

Back Exercises

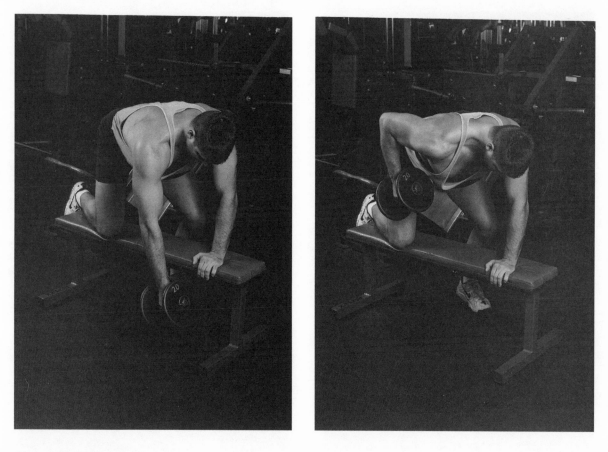

Dumbbell Rows

- Brace yourself on a bench with one hand as you bend over from the waist, letting the hand holding the dumbbell hang from your shoulder at arm's length.
- Keeping your back flat and your head up, lift the dumbbell to your side. Make sure the elbow is up and out, away from your body, contracting the muscles in the middle back.
- Lower the weight slowly and repeat on the other side. Try to use the back muscles, keeping involvement of your arm muscles to a minimum.

Back Exercises

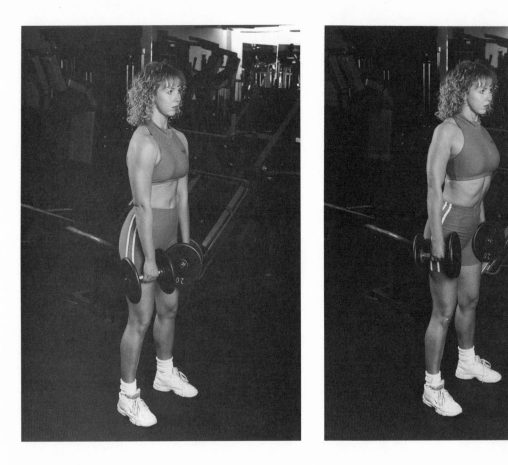

Shrugs

- These can be done with either the bar or the dumbbell.
- Stand with your torso straight, your hands at your sides holding the weight.
- Lift shoulders up and back, contracting the trapezius muscles of the upper back and neck.
- Hold in the top position for five seconds before releasing slowly to the original position.

Back Exercises

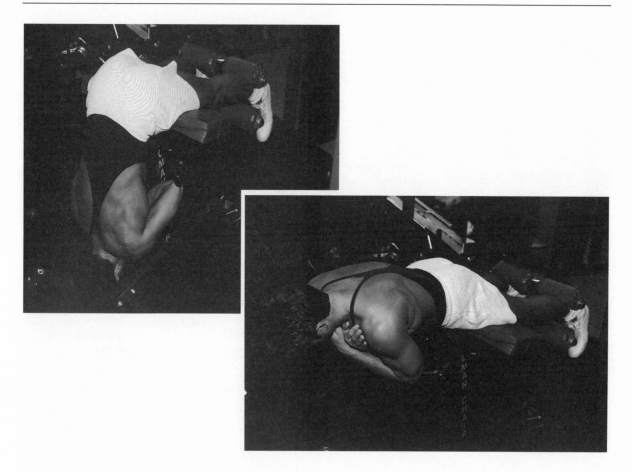

Hyper-Extensions

- Position your hips and hook your feet under the rollers or support bar.
- Cross your arms over your chest or clasp your hands behind your head, and lower your body.
- Do not swing back and forth, keep your back straight and steady as you return to the upright position.
- Concentrate on keeping the back flat and on working the spinal erector muscles of the lower back in this exercise.

Back Exercises

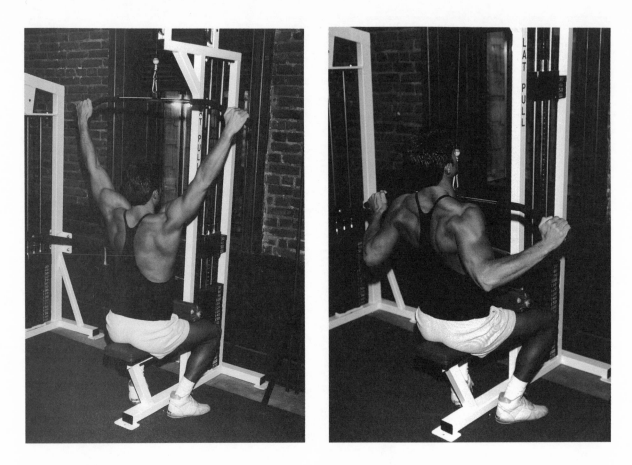

Lat Pulldown

- Sitting in the machine with your knees hooked under the support, keep your head up and your torso straight.
- Take the bar in a wide overhand grip and pull it down smoothly until it touches the top of your chest. During movement, keep your elbows well back, keeping the body from swaying back to involve your lower back.
- When you release, let the arms extend to give a full stretch to the latissimus dorsi muscles in the middle to lower part of the back.
- To emphasize the upper latissimus muscles, pull the bar down behind the neck.
- When doing either position, remember to keep your back straight and steady, your elbows leading back and away from the chest.

Back Exercises

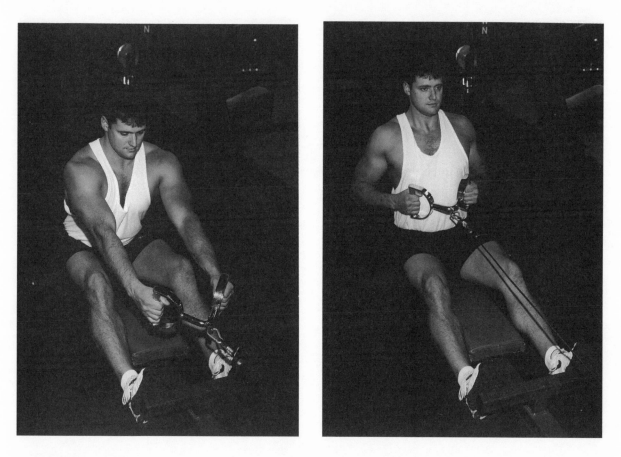

Long Cable Row

- Sitting in the machine with feet braced against the crossbar, keep your knees slightly bent and stretch forward to grasp cable handles.
- Pull back toward your body until you are sitting upright, not leaning backward.
- Push your chest out and draw your shoulder blades back while squeezing the bar to your abdomen.
- Keep the weight under control as you release it and let the bar go forward again.

Back Exercises

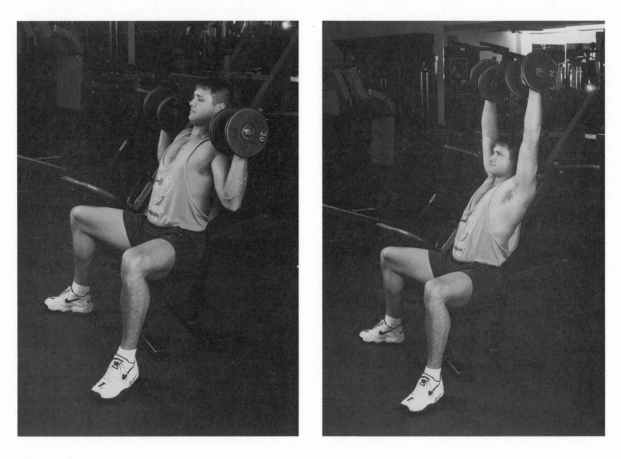

Military Press

- This exercise can be done either seated or standing, using dumbbells or a straight bar.
- Grasp the weight with your palms forward, your hands slightly more than shoulder width apart. If using a bar, position your hands far enough apart so that your arms maintain a 90-degree angle to the bar as you complete the movement of the exercise.
- Hold the weight at shoulder level and lift it straight overhead. Keep your back straight, lifting until you can lock your arms.
- Maintaining balance and control, lower the weight slowly back to the starting position.

Shoulder Exercises

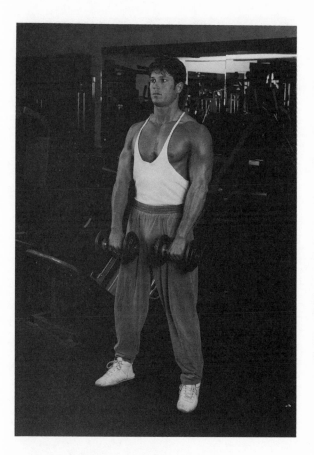 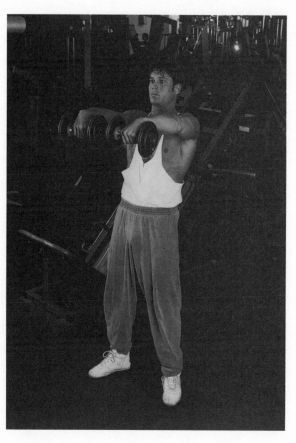

Front Dumbbell Raises

- This exercise can be done seated or standing, also with a straight bar.
- Keep your torso erect and your arms straight throughout the exercise.
- If using dumbbells, start with arms down, the weights in front of your thighs. With your wrists relaxed, raise weights to shoulder level.
- If using a barbell, begin by taking the bar in an overhand grip, hanging down in front of you at arm's length. Lift it to shoulder level, keeping your arms straight.
- Maintain controlled steady movements as you lower the weight.

Shoulder Exercises

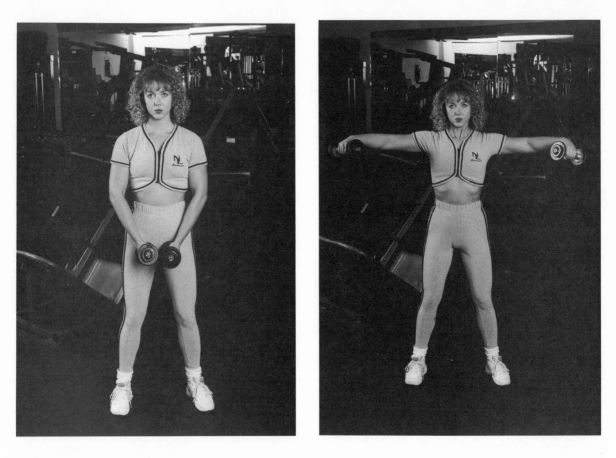

Lateral Dumbbell Raises

- This exercise can also be done on a cable machine.
- Keep your feet shoulder width apart and your elbows slightly bent as you take a dumbbell in each hand, bringing the weights together in front of you.
- With relaxed wrists, lift the weights out and up away from you to either side.
- After they reach shoulder level, lower the dumbbells slowly, maintaining control all the way down.
- This exercise can also be done alternating the arm movements.

Shoulder Exercises

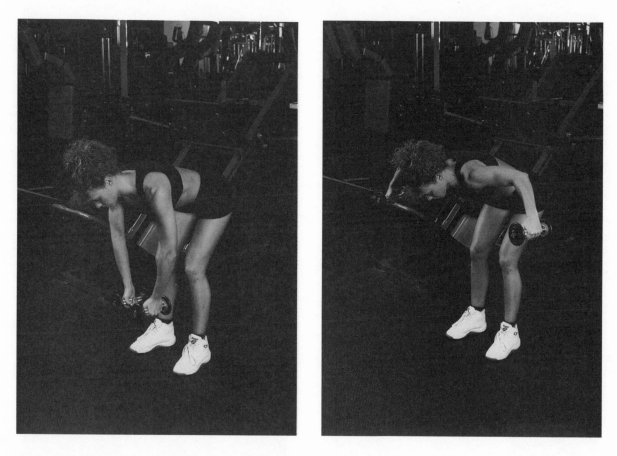

Rear Dumbbell, or Bent Lateral, Raises

- This exercise can be done seated or standing.
- Hold a dumbbell in each hand and bend from the waist, allowing the weights to hang at arm's length below you.
- With your back flat and your arms slightly bent, lift the weights up and out to the side until you reach shoulder level. Concentrate on contracting the rear of the deltoid muscles while doing this. Don't let the weights drift back as you raise them.
- Lower the weights slowly, resisting all the way down.

Shoulder Exercises

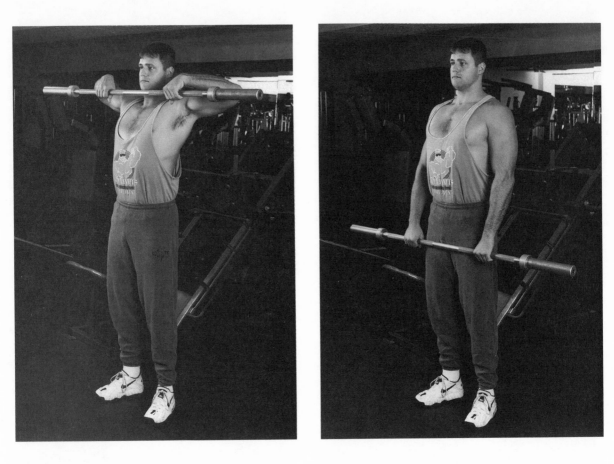

Upright Rows

- This exercise can be done with a bar, dumbbells, or cable.
- Standing with your hands less than shoulder width apart, in an overhand grip on the bar, let the bar hang at arm's length straight down in front of you.
- Keep your back straight and lift the bar straight up, close to the front of your body, until it comes to your chin. Your whole shoulder girdle should rise in a shrug, elbows above the bar.
- Lower the weight under control.

Shoulder Exercises

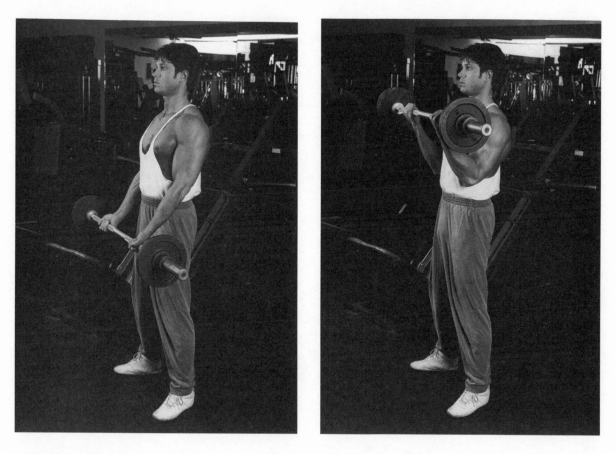

Barbell Curls

- Stand with your feet a few inches apart and grasp the barbell with an underhand grip, your hands shoulder width apart.
- Start with the bar hanging down at arm's length in front of you. Curl the weight out and up as high as you can, fully contracting the biceps.
- Lower the bar following the same arc, resisting the weight all the way back to the starting point.

Biceps and Forearm Exercises

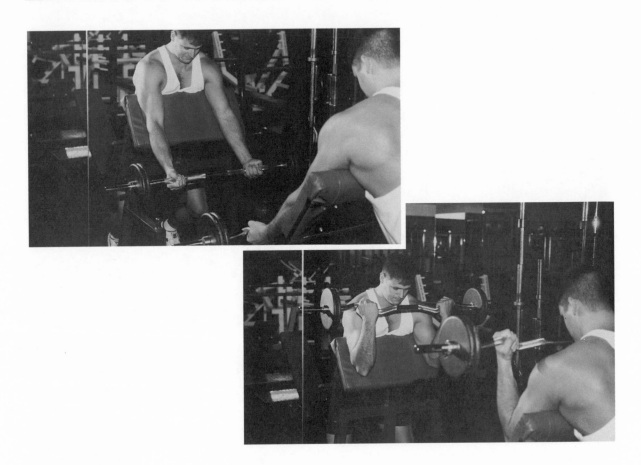

Preacher Curls

- This exercise can be done sitting or standing.
- Place your chest against the back pad of bench, with the arm extended over the pad. Grasp the barbell in an underhand grip.
- With your wrists locked, curl the bar up, holding the contraction for a few seconds at the top.
- Lower with control.

Biceps and Forearm Exercises

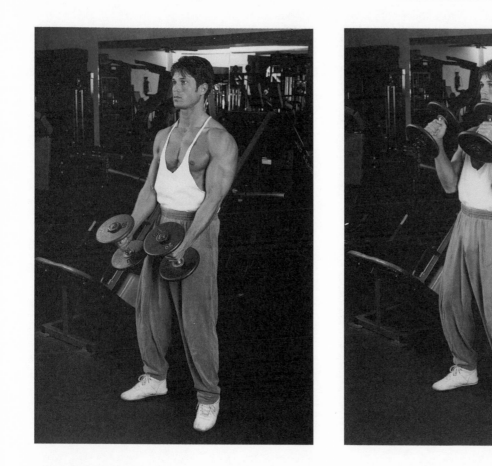

Hammer Curls

- Standing, with body straight and elbows locked at your sides, take a dumbbell in each hand with your palms facing each other, the dumbbell plates facing front.
- With your wrists locked, lift weights out and up.
- Lower weights slowly with control.
- In gripping the dumbbells, keep your thumbs up, facing ceiling.

Biceps and Forearm Exercises

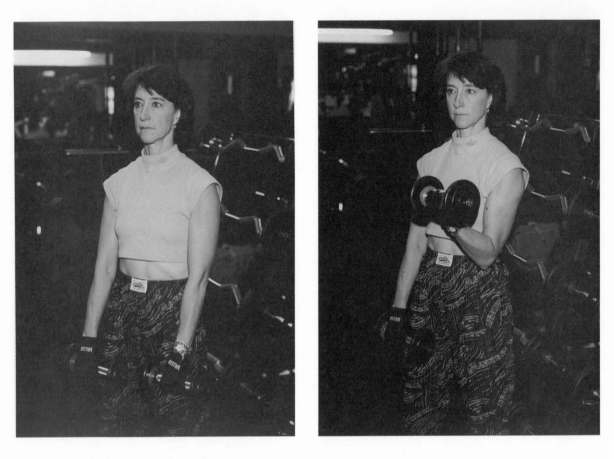

Alternating Dumbbell Curls

- This exercise can be done sitting or standing.
- Begin with a dumbbell in each hand, hanging at arm's length, with palms facing backward.
- Lift the weight with one hand, curling up and out, your arm close to your side.
- While you are lifting the weight, twist your wrist so that your palm ends facing forward at the finish.
- As you begin to lower one weight, simultaneously begin to raise the weight in the other arm, again twisting the wrists of both arms so that one palm ends up facing out, the other facing backward.
- Perform complete movements, slowly and under control.

Biceps and Forearm Exercises

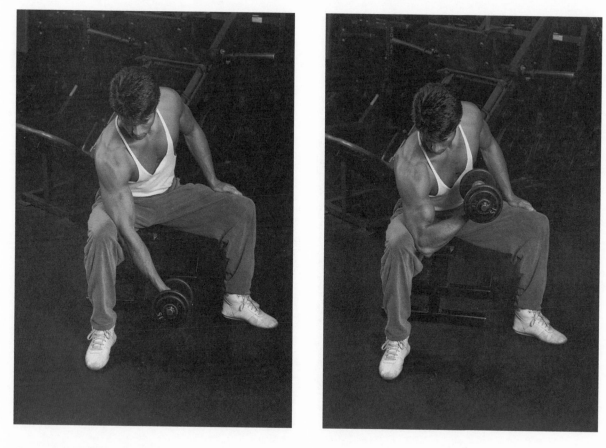

Concentration Curls

- In a sitting position, spread your knees, take hold of a dumbbell in one hand, and allow that arm to hang straight down inside the leg on its side. Place the elbow of the other arm on other leg.
- With the back of the hand facing the floor, raise the dumbbell without moving your upper arm or elbow.
- Do not use your leg to support the elbow of your lifting arm; just use the leg as a guide for positioning the arm.
- As you lift, twist your wrist so that the back of your lifting hand, which started facing the floor, ends up facing the ceiling.
- Alternate arms.

Biceps and Forearm Exercises

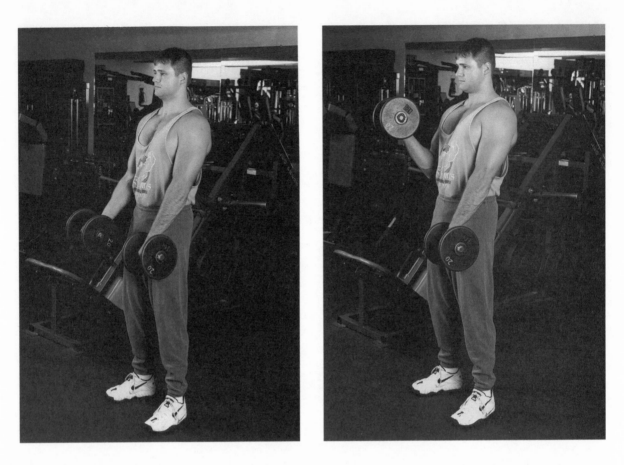

Zottman Curls

- This exercise can be done sitting or standing.
- Begin with the dumbbells in each hand, your arms straight and your palms facing backward.
- Keep your arms close at your sides as you curl the dumbbells up. Twist your wrists so that at the top of the lift, you have your palms upward.
- Lower your arms slowly in control, again twisting your wrists to end with your palms downward.

Biceps and Forearm Exercises

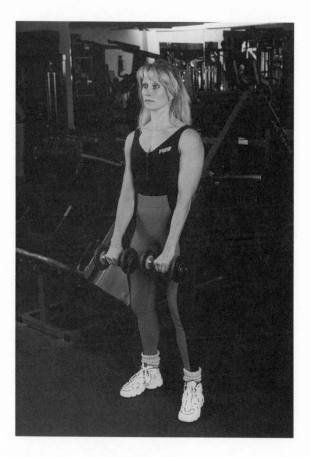 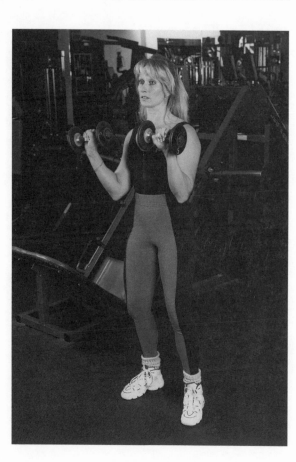

Reverse Dumbbell Curls

- Use shoulder-width grip on dumbbells, palms down.
- Standing, keep your body straight and your feet shoulder width apart as you let the dumbbells hang down in front of you.
- Keep your elbows and your upper arms in at your sides as you curl dumbbells up.

Biceps and Forearm Exercises

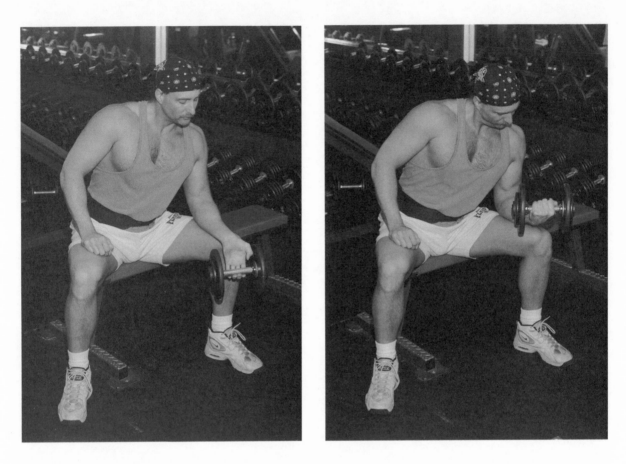

Barbell Wrist Curls

- This exercise can also use dumbbells.
- Seated, take hold of the dumbbell with an underhand grip, your forearm resting on top of your thigh.
- Flex your wrist and lower the weight toward the floor, then lift it back to the starting point, keeping your forearms steady.

Biceps and Forearm Exercises

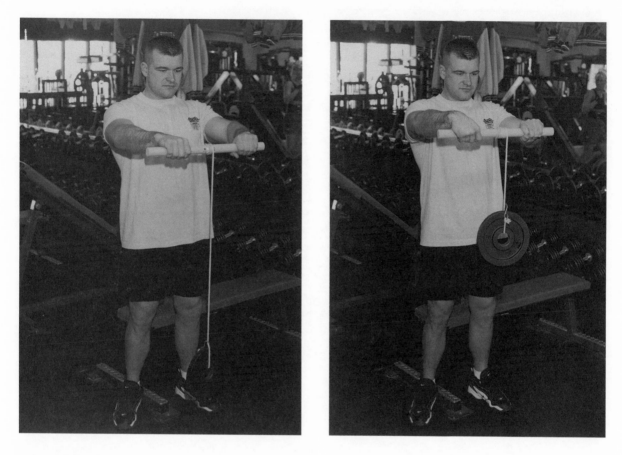

Rope Twist

- Perform with the weight tied to a short bar with about three feet of rope.
- Take hold of the bar using both hands. Twist bar to roll up weight.

Biceps and Forearm Exercises

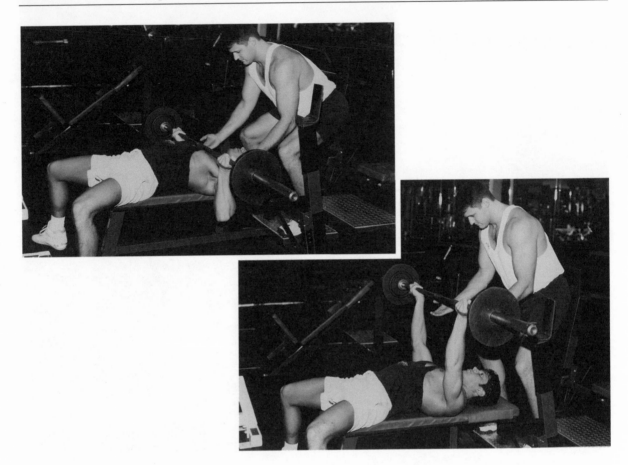

Reverse Grip Bench Press

- Lie on the bench and grip the bar with your palms facing you.
- Lift the bar off the rack and lower it slowly, return it to the rack in control. Do not bounce the bar.
- Select grip position according to your sticking point in the bench press: stick low, off chest—use wide grip; stick high, top end—use close grip; stick midway—use grip midway between wide and close.

Triceps Exercises

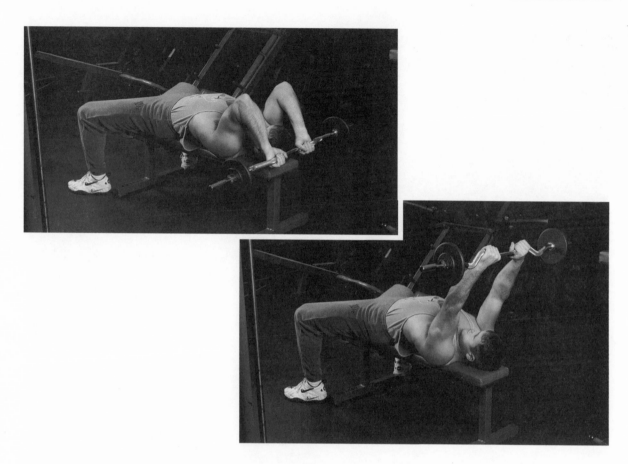

Lying Triceps Extensions, or French Curls

- Lie along a bench, and using an overhand grip, take hold of a barbell.
- Use a narrow grip on the bar, with your thumbs about mid–shoulder width.
- Begin by pressing the weight up and out behind your head, arms locking at about a 45-degree angle.
- Keeping the elbows stationary, lower weight by bending down toward the top of your head.
- Press back to the starting position, all the time feeling the work in your triceps.

Triceps Exercises

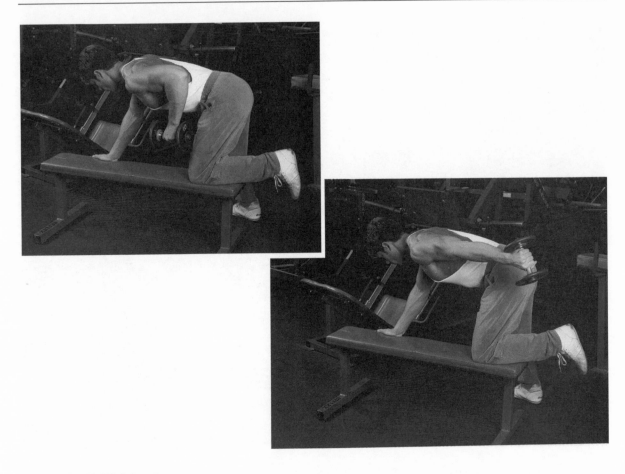

Dumbbell Kickbacks

- Using a bench to support one hand, bend at the waist so your back is parallel to the floor.
- Take a dumbbell in your other hand, raising your elbow back and up to shoulder height. Keep your upper arm and elbow in fixed positions tight against your side, while your forearm hangs straight down toward the floor.
- Without moving the elbow, slowly raise the weight back until your arm is fully out, parallel to the floor.
- After holding a moment to feel contraction in your triceps, slowly lower your forearm back to a downward position. Only your forearm moves in this exercise.

Triceps Exercises

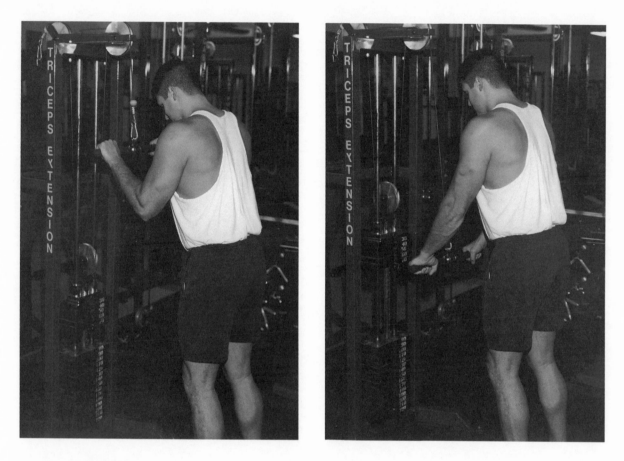

Cable Pushdowns

- Stand close to the bar and take it with an overhand grip with arms bent at a 45-degree angle in the up position.
- Keep your upper arms and elbows in fixed positions tight against your sides as you push the bar down toward the floor as far as possible with your forearms. Release and let the bar come up as far as possible, again without moving your upper arms and elbows.
- Keep your body straight during this exercise; do not lean as you push down. Keep your chest expanded.
- This exercise can also be done with a single handle.

Triceps Exercises

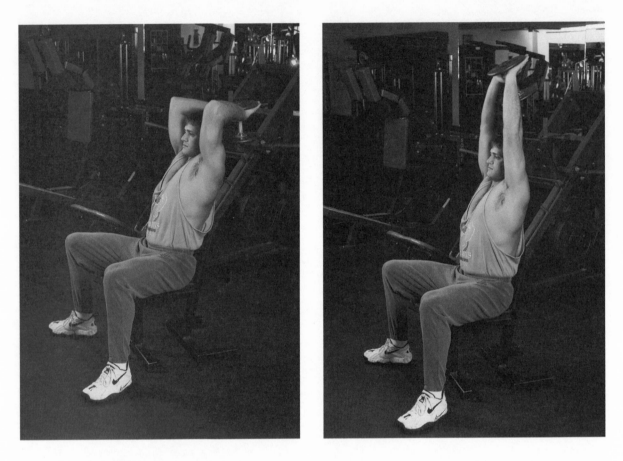

Seated Dumbbell Extensions

- Hold a single dumbbell behind head, palms pressed under the top plate, using both hands palms up.
- Sit on a bench, your feet flat on the floor, and raise the dumbbell straight over your head.
- Keep your upper arms and elbows stationary, close to your ears.
- Lower the dumbbell directly behind your head, as far as possible for the stretch.
- Now, using your triceps, raise the dumbbell back over your head to the full extension. All the movement should be in the forearms; keep your upper arms and elbows stationary.

Triceps Exercises

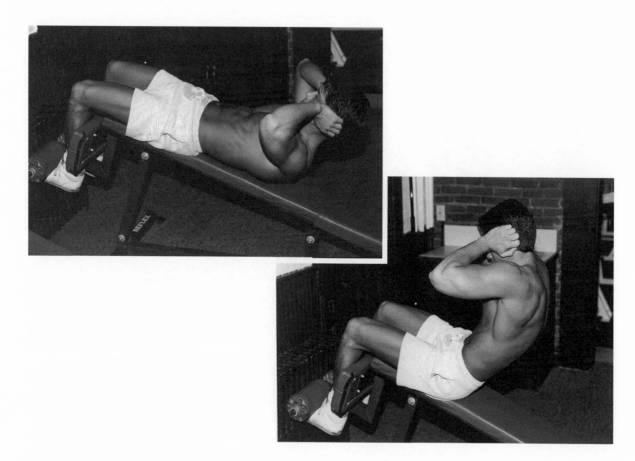

Crunches

- This exercise can be done on a slant board or on the floor.
- Lie on the floor with bent knees, your feet flat on floor, or rest your calves over a bench.
- Cross your arms over your chest and lift your shoulders up by contracting your abdominal muscles toward your hips.
- Do not pull on your neck or place your hands at the sides of your head.
- Squeeze your stomach in toward your spine as you bend, keeping your lower back pressed against the floor throughout the exercise.
- Concentrate on using the abdominal muscles to lift and lower, keeping your legs relaxed.
- Exhale as you lift and bend forward; inhale as you release and lower yourself back to the floor.

NOTE: Don't be too rigid about the number of reps you give to abdominal exercises. If you do them regularly, your progress will be quick. There is no need to risk getting an injury.

Abdominal Exercises

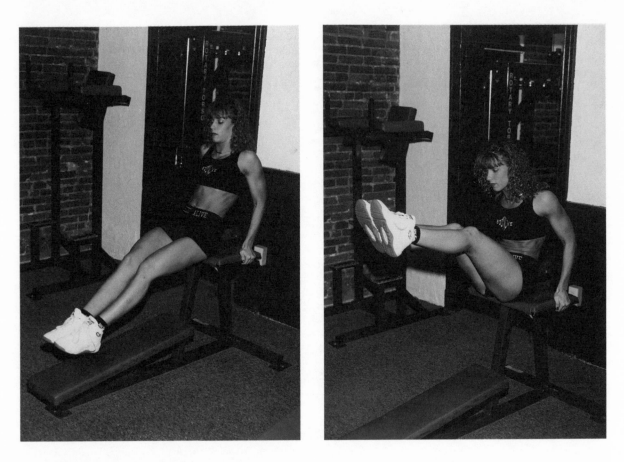

Seated Leg Raises, or Leg Tucks

- Sit with your buttocks on the edge of a flat bench, and, holding on to the edge for support, angle your body back at about 45 degrees. At the same time, pull your abdominals in toward your spine.
- Keep your legs extended out, your knees slightly bent, with feet approximately four inches off the floor.
- Exhale while lifting your feet in a sweeping motion toward the ceiling, bringing your legs up as far as you can.
- Inhale while lowering your feet to your original position.

Abdominal Exercises

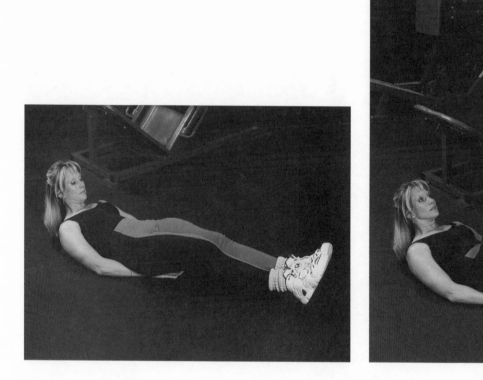

Incline Leg Raises

- Lie on the floor with your knees slightly bent and your feet about four inches off the floor. Place your hands under your hips for support.
- Squeeze your abdominals toward your spine and exhale as you start each rep.
- Exhaling, raise your feet up and over your hips.
- Press your heels toward the ceiling, lifting your hips off the floor using your abdominal muscles.
- Inhaling, slowly lower your feet back to the original position without arching your back. If you can't stop yourself from arching your back, or otherwise have trouble with the lift, increase the bend in your knees until your abs are stronger.

Abdominal Exercises

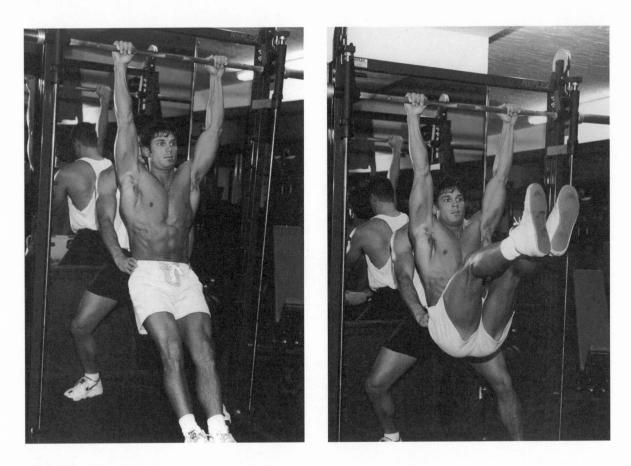

Hanging Leg Raises

- Raise your arms up and take hold of a pull-up bar with an overhand grip, your hands shoulder width apart.
- Rotate your hips and draw your legs up toward the ceiling, with your knees fixed in a slightly bent position. At the same time, strongly squeeze your abdominals.
- Do not swing from the bar; keep your back rounded.
- Lower your legs slowly and with control. Do not bend your legs back too far; you should always be able to see your feet in this exercise.

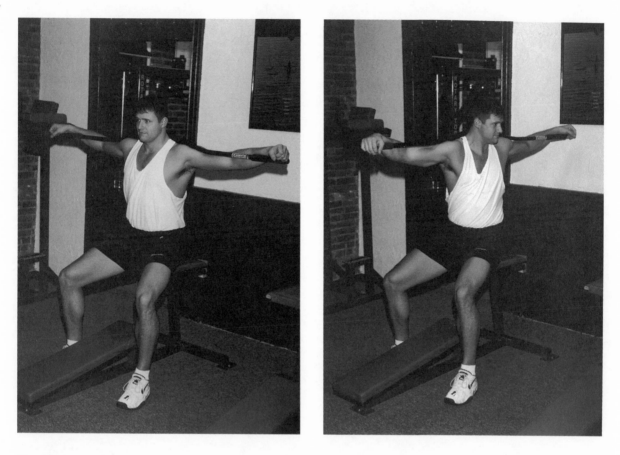

Twists

- Hold a light bar or broom handle behind your neck with both hands.
- Keep your back straight, your feet flat on the floor, and your hips forward.
- While the rest of your body is kept steady, twist from the waist first to one side, then the other as far as you can go. During the twist, concentrate on working the oblique muscles at either side of your abdominals and the muscles around your ribs.
- This exercise can be done seated or standing.

Abdominal Exercises

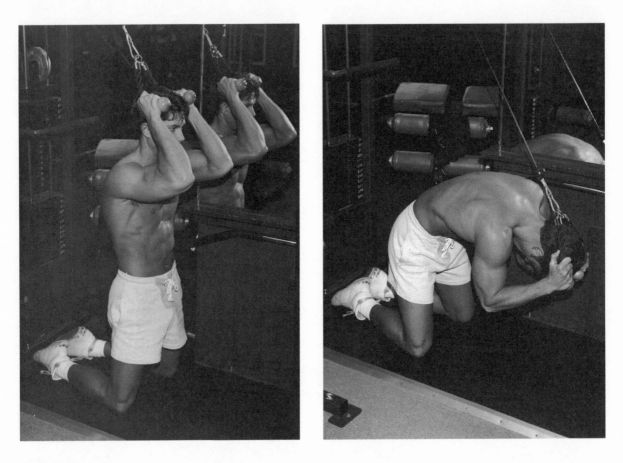

Cable Crunches

- Attach a rope extension to an upper cable. With your back to the cable, kneel on the floor with the rope held at forehead level.
- Keep your thighs perpendicular to the floor. Do not sit back on your heels during this exercise.
- Holding the rope, contract your abdominals and pull your elbows halfway down to your knees.
- This exercise can be done to the front or alternating side to side.

Abdominal Exercises

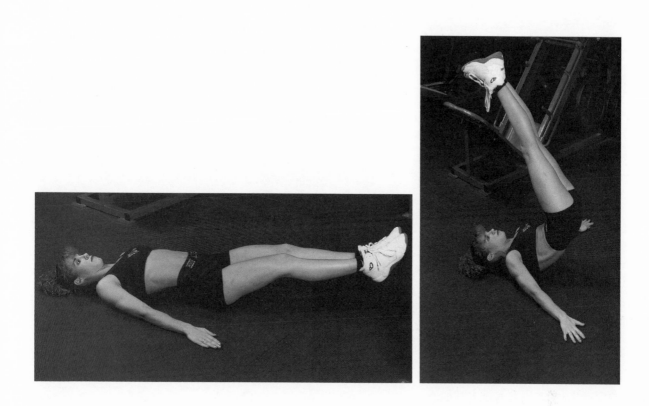

Knee Lifts

- Lie on the floor with your knees slightly bent, your feet flat on floor.
- With your arms straight out and your palms on the floor, lift your feet off the floor and lead with them until your lower back lifts off the floor.
- Return to the original position without letting your feet touch the floor.

Abdominal Exercises

Chapter Fourteen

The Ultimate Motivation

If you are reading this book, you probably have at least some vague desire to improve your health and your life. The good thing about desires is that they can lead us to new and valuable experiences. The trouble with them is that they are often vague and hard to hold on to, even when they involve matters that are very important to us. If you want to find out whether your desire for a better life is one you don't want to let get away, test it.

The best way to do that is to see if you can turn it into a vision of yourself. Visions aren't made up of the casual stuff of desires; they get deep inside your hopes for yourself and inside your belief in yourself. They are clear, completely grounded in reality, and very powerful. If you find that you are able to picture down to the smallest details what it will be like when you have a lean, strong body, you can make it happen.

The reason for this is that goals come from visions. Clear, attainable goals focus your efforts and guide your decisions. Goals keep you steady and patient when there are setbacks. Having a vision for yourself also puts a special energy into your efforts and your will. This energy is often called commitment. Commitment means you can keep working toward what you want whether everything is going your way or not. Clear goals and commitment together bring success, success being the ultimate motivation.

Index

Visit John's web site at

www.the-factor.com

For your nutritional needs, John has arranged a great discount for his readers
on a full line of nutritional supplement products manufactured by an
FDA-approved facility, with absolute guaranteed quality.
For product information, call toll free 1-800-222-3339.